Managing Information and Knowledge in the Public Sector

For the public sector, which is globally the largest employer of people and repository of information, managing information and knowledge is an extremely problematic area to address. The essence of both resources is that they are intangible – their impact and value cannot be measured through traditional accounting methods – yet they are also, paradoxically, where the greatest value and potential for improvement is located. In this book Eileen Milner introduces the reader to the concepts of information and knowledge and explores a variety of tools and techniques which may be usefully adopted in actively managing and developing these resources. Wherever possible, real-life public sector cases and examples are used to illustrate good practice, as well as some of the pitfalls of poor application. Down-to-earth and taking into account the critically important characteristics unique to public services, this will be an illuminating text both for managers and policy makers already working in the public sector and for those considering doing so.

Eileen Milner is a Principal Lecturer in Information Management at the University of North London.

Managing Information and Knowledge in the Public Sector

Eileen M. Milner

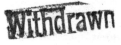

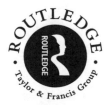

London and New York

First published 2000
by Routledge
11 New Fetter Lane, London EC4P 4EE

Simultaneously published in the USA and Canada
by Routledge
29 West 35th Street, New York, NY 10001

Routledge is an imprint of the Taylor & Francis Group

Typeset in Times by Taylor & Francis Books Ltd
Printed and bound in Great Britain by Biddles Ltd,
Guildford and King's Lynn

British Library Cataloguing in Publication Data
A catalogue record for this book is available from the British Library

Library of Congress Cataloging in Publication Data
Milner, Eileen M., 1963–
   Managing information and knowledge in the public sector/
   Eileen M. Milner.
   p.cm.
   Includes bibliographical references and index.
   1. Knowledge management. 2. Information
   technology–Management. 3. Organizational learning.
   4. Information capitol. I. Title.
HD30.2 .M54 2000
352.3'8–dc21   00-020795

ISBN 0–415–20422–4 (hbk)
ISBN 0–415–20423–2 (pbk)

This book is dedicated to the memory of Margaret and Joe Milner

Contents

Preface

A number of factors came together to persuade me, in 1997, that there was a need for a publication that addressed itself specifically to issues of information and knowledge management in the public sector. By then, as an information management specialist with a primary interest in the concept of developing valuation methodologies for information and knowledge assets, I had had the opportunity (more by chance than foresight and planning) to lead important research into the development of what is most often referred to as 'electronic government'. This research considered practice in the UK, Europe, Singapore, Canada, the United States and Australia, and what I found was disquieting to say the least: for public sector organisations seemed to have embraced the promises of information and communications technologies with almost profligate enthusiasm, with little evidence that the quality and structure of services being delivered had been significantly enhanced, or that end-user satisfaction rates had been significantly improved.

Thus, the need for a text that focused on achieving some meaningful synthesis around issues of information and knowledge management for a public sector audience grew and evolved from a research context that showed these to be all-pervasive as *terms* in the lexicon of public sector reform, but almost invisible when actual application and implementation of change agenda were explored. From the outset, it has been the author's goal to achieve a text which is both rigorous and theoretically defensible in its approach to these complex issues, while at the same time striving to ensure that the work is accessible and relevant to as wide an audience of academics and practitioners – and indeed aspiring practitioners – as possible. Inevitably some degree of tension has emerged from lack of absolute convergence between these two aspirations: where it has, the decision has usually been to curtail emphasis upon an overly theoretical exploration of key issues and to focus instead upon maximising the potential for learning through analysis of actual practice.

However, it should be noted that there has been no neglect of matters theoretical by the author; rather, decisions around textual emphasis have sought to add clarity in an area where little sector-specific work has taken place to date around the synthesis of information and knowledge management issues. Yet this is not to deny the critical foundation works in related areas, particularly those of information policy, where key theoretical and conceptual frameworks have been provided by Taylor and Bellamy, Feather and Dutton; these writers make a valuable contribution to arriving at a perspective on whether information and knowledge represent the greatest area of collective waste and neglect, or conversely the greatest opportunity for achieving the full potential for reform, within public sector structures.

Of course, it is right to acknowledge that organisations in the public sector are subject to a range of environmental factors – such as complex issues of accountability, changing political agendas and a perceived absence of an underlying profit motive – not usually associated with the commercial sector, where so much of the focus upon issues of information and knowledge management has so far taken place. However, it is appropriate to ask whether they are really that different in terms of how the public sector operates. Is there a danger that difference, or at least perceived difference, becomes instead an excuse for the failure and inertia in these areas which seems to prevail to such a large extent today? This climate is changing, and it is changing rapidly, but as we shall explore in almost every chapter of this book, it remains one where senior managers and politicians have become enamoured of the 'soundbite' that is information and knowledge management and seem ready to embrace the rhetoric without fully understanding the basic principles, requirements and responsibilities which are essential to achieving success in this area.

Therefore, the underpinning premise of this book is that, too often, issues of 'difference' are used to excuse both the inertia and some elements of failure to achieve anticipated improvements on investment, particularly in information and communications technologies (ICTs). The term 'dinosaur' is often used disparagingly, by politicians particularly, to describe the operating culture which they perceive to be dominant in the public sector. Yet, if one seeks an alternative metaphor to describe what it is that the public sector should be aspiring to, there is little evidence from either the literature – or indeed from commentators – that this has been articulated as being anything more than the need to strive to be more 'modern', and more 'flexible'. However, a focus upon issues of information and knowledge management does suggest a strategic vision which sees the public sector as being less like a dinosaur and more like a dolphin – inasmuch as we are seeking to chart a path to a position of service design and delivery, which is *intelligent, agile, keen* and *able to learn, accomplished at communication* and ultimately, perhaps, *likeable* for those who engage with it.

However, setting aside the author's own original motivation and indeed occasional frustration with public sector structures and applications, there are, of course, very important issues underpinning the discussion of information and knowledge management which require serious and ongoing attention by all areas of the 'public sector'. Most critically, the approach adopted and advocated here is one which emphasises the almost symbiotic relationship between information and knowledge. Too often, both academics and practitioners fall into a potentially dangerous outlook which artificially separates information from knowledge and knowledge from information, neglecting to focus upon the fact that information is frequently the nourishment of knowledge creation and may itself be a by-product of the knowledge generation process. It is therefore the intention of this text to make some small contribution to the emergence of both debate and practice in this critical area, in a 'joined-up' and coherent manner focusing upon issues which, as we shall see in subsequent chapters, if properly addressed are capable of making a significant and lasting impact upon what is actually meant by the 'public sector'.

Eileen Milner

Acknowledgements

When originally putting forward the case for what is essentially the first major text on the management of information and knowledge assets in the public sector, I thought the major scale of the undertaking was apparent. However, over the year in which this work has been in progress, I have had to revise upwards my own views of the complexity of the subject area under discussion, particularly with the ever-greater pace of change in reforming public services within the framework of what are commonly termed the 'information society' and the 'knowledge economy'. I have also had opportunity to commend the far-sightedness of my publishers, Routledge, and of the commissioning editor for this text, Heather Gibson, who at the outset of this project had little evidence, beyond their own instinct, that the concepts of information and knowledge management were likely to move centre-stage in a global context in the reform of public services.

Where at all possible, examples drawn from real-life practice have been used to illustrate key concepts discussed within the text. The examples used have sought to highlight practice outside both the United States and the European Union, the reasons for this being twofold: first, to acknowledge that excellent practice is emerging globally, and second, to attempt to overcome, in the mind of the user of this text, any of the latent geographic prejudice which is often discernible when discussing examples of what might be loosely termed 'emerging best practice'. Indeed, in my experience as a European national who has conducted research in this area in both Europe and North America, there is an underlying reluctance in both populations to engage in meaningful learning and development exercises which involve possible adoption of practices between and across national and regional boundaries. Thus, to overcome this at least in part, it will be noted at an early stage that when offering pointers to generalisable developments much use is made of practice found in Australia, a country which, perhaps because of its location and history, can be viewed as reasonably neutral. However, perhaps even more important, the example of Australia deserves on its own merit to receive a place of prominence in a text dealing with issues of information and knowledge management, as it has probably one of the best-developed approaches to harnessing such assets in a drive to reform the way in which the public sector is structured to 'do business'. Therefore, I must express my gratitude to the many public service workers in Australia to whom I am indebted for both their hospitality and their patience during my extended visit to the country, and who have continued to support me through helpful briefings since then. However, a particular word of thanks must be directed to Sarah Brasch, who has been a true friend to this project, and also to Helen Ringrose, who facilitated such a beneficial visit to Brisbane.

I am grateful too to colleagues who spend their lives observing the nuances of the public sector and of information and knowledge management (IKM) more generally. Among these are Alan Burkitt-Gray and Marcus Pollett, the editorial team on *Government Computing*, both of whom have been supportive and unstinting in their willingness to share observations and emerging news with me. Thanks too must go to Graham Coult, the editor of *Managing Information*, whose support, advice and friendship has sustained me through the many times when completion of this book seemed to be nothing more than a distant aspiration. And to Nigel Oxbrow and Angela Abell from TFPL, thanks too, for their willingness to share their considerable knowledge of emerging best practice with me and for opening up opportunities to discuss issues of importance to this text with practitioners from the commercial sectors.

Within my own institution, the University of North London, I have been grateful for the friendship, support and patience of many colleagues. Particular thanks are due to Roy Williams and his team within Information Systems and Services, particularly Ann Aungle and her colleagues in the library who have been so supportive of searches for rather obscure references. Thanks are due also to the team of postgraduate staff and students with whom I work, who have provided me with many thought-provoking and challenging opportunities for reflection. Within this context, particular thanks must be given to Elena Moschini, who has shown such patience with my often inept attempts at explanation of technical issues.

More formally, thanks and acknowledgement must be attributed to the Stationery Office, the Australian Department of the Prime Minister and to IMPACT Ltd, each of whom promptly and willingly provided permission for reproduction of their copyright materials.

Finally, it is in the gift of most authors to publicly record their debts of gratitude to those who have personally supported them through the often tortuous and lonely stages of writing a sole-authored text. Thus, it is important to record my gratitude to Breda Hanrahan, Daisy and Kathleen Sinnott and Margaret and Joan Cullen, Gillian Cloke and Andrew Hodge, as well, of course, as Catherine, Verity and Edward, for providing treasured levels of friendship and support during often difficult times. Pat and Gerald Atkinson have been always on hand with support and practical help, as well as undoubted care and concern which has never been more appreciated. Brigid Milner has been a key figure in motivating me to keep writing; as a sister and an academic critic, she is precious indeed. And final thanks go to my husband Richard Atkinson, for whom there are insufficient words to express my gratitude for his patience and support.

Chapter 1

Introduction

Defining information and knowledge

A key challenge for *any* organisation in the twenty-first century is to seek to maintain and improve its performance in an increasingly complex and competitive global operating environment, where change pressures appear to offer the only certainty. Despite the pursuit, over the last two decades, of 'Total Quality Management' (TQM), 'Business Process Reengineering' (BPR) and more recently 'Enterprise Resource Planning' (ERP), to name only three of the more popular management holy grails, there remains, nonetheless, a prevailing sense of failure in fully realising hoped-for levels of improvement. In this context then, it is not surprising that there should be some sense of cynicism when it is argued that, by focusing upon identifying, valuing and managing information and knowledge (IKM) assets, there are significant opportunities to achieve more effective organisations and to improve their efficiency by reducing the amount of wasted time, effort and lost opportunity through better and more integrated use of both *tangible* and *intangible* organisational resources. The challenge presented here is to move to define such assets, particularly in relation to a 'public sector' context, and through an investigation of the benefits which can accrue from the successful management of information and knowledge, to dispel much of the disquiet and cynicism surrounding this potentially important area of organisational improvement.

Thus, during the course of this text our challenge is to explore what information and knowledge assets actually are, and then to consider strategies for managing them within the particular range of contexts that represent the diverse modern interpretation of the 'public sector'. To do this is in itself a complex undertaking, for the identification and management of such assets represents a significant challenge. As both a theoretical concept and a management application, such an approach is intrinsically problematic, for what you are attempting to give structure and assign value to is very often *intangible*: by its very nature it involves people and their behaviour with regard to information and knowledge generation and use.

Such essentially dynamic processes do not readily lend themselves to analysis by traditional accounting methods, nor do they necessarily sit comfortably within established legal frameworks, particularly in respect of issues of intellectual property and the legal admissibility of electronically generated and stored documentation. However, just as in the 1980s when, primarily because of the trend towards large-scale mergers and acquisitions, overwhelming business pressures forced commercial sector organisations to begin to focus on the importance and financial value of their brands, the opening years of the twenty-first century represent a similarly defining moment, in the recognition that information and knowledge assets are potentially key contributors to the achievement of improvement. Therefore, our underpinning premise is that any cynicism generated by the introduction of what might be characterised as yet another management fad is likely to be dispelled, or at least tempered, upon more enlightened understanding of the scope and importance of the management of information and knowledge in an applied organisational context. In order to do this successfully a number of deceptively straightforward principles must be understood, which acknowledge that:

- within organisations there is an imperative for the data generation process to be understood;
- data gathering and organisation for use and extraction of value should then become a priority;
- 'data' is transformed into information through appropriate dissemination and interpretation;
- information, when used appropriately, assists in knowledge generation and decision-making processes;
- the culmination of the data to information to knowledge process is the creation of organisational 'wisdom', the accumulation of learning processes that help successful organisations to move forward.

During the course of subsequent chapters, each of these elements will be discussed both theoretically and in relation to operational contexts where their integration as processes can be said to illustrate both the benefits and the difficulties of moving towards the development of an IKM-focused organisation.

The term 'information and knowledge management' (IKM) is in itself an important one, important not only in respect of what we will later discover it capable of achieving in an applied context, but theoretically critical in respect of the linkage that it assumes, as outlined above, between information and knowledge. The simple model, represented in Figure 1.1, from data generation through to information creation, interpretation and use, knowledge sharing and perhaps ultimately judgement and wisdom, is one that we shall explore in greater detail in subsequent chapters. It represents the intellectual and applied foundations of this emerging academic and professional discipline, and is essentially an holistic view, incorporating strategic and operational issues as well as making explicit linkages to areas such as systems analysis and processing, communications and marketing functions, and financial and human resource management. To undertake IKM requires that an organisation be aware of the data/information/knowledge processes currently operating within it, and be capable of and committed to improving the efficacy of these processes through the use of appropriate tools and techniques which emphasise the intertwined goals of achieving *collection* and *connection*.

Some of the 'tools' mentioned above are the information and communications technologies (ICTs), without the development of which the potential offered by IKM would only ever be partially fulfilled. However, from the outset it is critical to assign these technologies to their proper place in the IKM continuum, and that is very much a supporting and enabling position. Taken together with the fact that senior managers within all types of organisations were (and perhaps the majority continue to be) largely inexpert in their understanding of ICT applications and their organisational implications, the rapid development in the capabilities of ICTs has led to huge investments in ICTs, made globally by all types of organisation, that fail to bring about significant return upon the investment made. In fact, a 1996 research report produced by Mori suggested that some 90 per cent of such investment was so poorly focused upon organisational requirements that it failed to contribute to operating or strategic improvements (Mori 1996). Further, Madrick cautions in his review of the US economy that:

> Far from increasing productivity gains, the increasing use of computer technology actually slows them down … Business has increased its investment in computers by more than 30 per cent a year since the early 1970s but the rate of growth of productivity has fallen from 2.85 per cent a year between 1947 and 1973 to about 1.1 per cent a year since 1973.
>
> (cited in May 1998: 21)

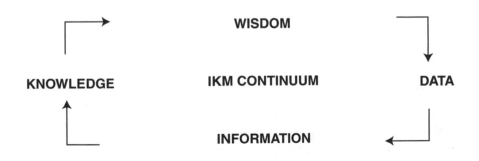

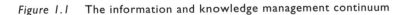

Figure 1.1   The information and knowledge management continuum

If we consider this in the context of the public sector, the focus for this study of IKM, we can begin to appreciate that globally it is possible, perhaps even likely, that large quantities of public finance have been used in such a manner, since the dash towards the achievement of what is sometimes referred to as 'electronic government' has been pursued with much enthusiasm. As Bird argues: 'Too often they [senior managers and politicians] fall in love with a technological innovation that has no practical use in the real world' (Bird 1996: 78).

Thus it can be observed that ICTs have powerful seductive charms for senior business executives and indeed for politicians. Sometimes their promise is fulfilled, too often it is not: automating a process or function, if that function is not structured appropriately or is in fact not what is required by the organisation or its customers, is not going to improve performance. So, for example, it was interesting to note that in the United Kingdom, during the 1998 celebrations of the fiftieth anniversary of the creation of the National Health Service, Prime Minister Tony Blair highlighted the perceived importance of telemedicine by granting it additional funding for development. While it is too soon to make any qualitative judgements and there is no intention to belittle the potential contribution of this area of health-care development, the question deserves to be raised as to whether this area was prioritised because it represented a key area of strategic priority and development for the UK's health service, or because the 'cutting edge' associations with ICTs were attractive to both politicians and media alike. This question of appropriate investment in technology and the critical importance of ensuring a linkage to wider strategic and operational issues is one that we shall return to many times during our exploration of IKM, reflecting some of the concerns raised by Davenport, who observes: 'While millions of high-tech entrepreneurs and bureaucrats work 16-hour days to improve information technology, virtually no one works on information behaviour and effect' (Davenport 1996: 10).

Setting aside the myths

It is important, then, to dispel at the outset the first of a number of myths that surround IKM: that it is a term that can be used variously as a direct substitute for 'information systems', 'information technology' or perhaps even 'decision support systems'. Certainly the ICT element of seeking to manage information and knowledge is an important one, and the competencies required of information and knowledge managers must encompass some level of technological understanding so that they are capable of outlining to technical experts what they need in terms of tasks required. However, too often, particularly when issues of information management (IM) are discussed, it is assumed that they are subsumed within ICT strategies and plans.

It is perhaps the apparent complexity of the processes associated with IKM that has led to a great deal of the confusion around what it actually is, and to the tendency to define it within terms that are more tangible, especially in regard to technology and related applications. The model of information and knowledge management that has been introduced in this chapter is essentially a continuum that represents the relationship between processes: it is an ideal, something that organisations should be working towards but which, as yet, very few have achieved.

As we will see when discussing specific aspects of IKM in greater detail in subsequent chapters, it is certainly possible to identify exemplars of good practice for a variety of aspects of the continuum. The greatest difficulty that we have at present is in identifying an example where sufficient maturity of practice has evolved to represent the holistic or 'joined-up' view of IKM that is desirable. This should not be viewed in an overly negative way, for rather than being solely an indicator of the difficulty of operationalising IKM strategies, it is perhaps better viewed as a pointer to the fact that the journey towards managing information and knowledge is never going to represent a 'quick fix': it is something that can only be achieved over time. In order to be successful it must impact upon the culture of the organisation, critically on the way in which *people* work and relate to one another and on the way in which these processes are organised to maximise their potential contribution to leveraging performance. Information and communications technologies can certainly play their part in the achievement of such effective information and knowledge management processes, but only as tools that underpin the achievement of organisation-wide strategies which, like the proverbial spider's web, link the management of information and knowledge assets to almost all aspects of operations and future planning.

When seeking to define the parameters of IKM, it is also important to consider the very real disquiet that can be generated when discussing IKM among those who view it as potentially having 'sinister' overtones. Indeed, academics who specialise in this area have been known to have had the light-hearted charge levelled against them that they are actually in the business of advocating the manipulation of information, particularly that which is intended for public consumption. Managing knowledge has the potential for also being seriously and sometimes mischievously misunderstood, with connotations of thought- and mind-control being put forward by many who do not appreciate the important organisational contribution that can be made by harnessing and formalising the sharing of colleagues' experiences and thinking on particular projects/tasks/functions. Such sinister connotations are not, of course, the case: the information and knowledge management processes that are discussed here in relation to organisational applications, particularly regarding the public sector, are those which seek to make most appropriate and efficient use of key resources and to ensure that they enhance the overall efficiency and effectiveness of the organisation, particularly in the way in which it interfaces with its customers, be they internal or external.

Once more, terminology has been unhelpful to the cause of IKM, for it is the case, in many public sector organisations particularly, that media and public relations activity is led by public employees with titles such as Information Officer or, still more confusingly, Information Manager. Misleading, manipulating or being otherwise economical with the truth in internal or public fora should have no place in IKM, the role of which is to ensure that key decision-makers, including communities of end-users where appropriate, have the benefit of appropriate information and accumulated knowledge prior to making a judgement and/or decision. The quality of outcome or intent underpinning such judgements is something for which the discipline of IKM should not be held directly accountable.

There are, additionally, significant problems which can arise from the use of the term 'management' itself. During the course of the author's own research into issues of IKM in the public sector, a recurring theme has been the extent to which senior managers, in a diverse range of public sector organisations, have railed against the use of this term 'management', particularly as associated with commercial sector paradigms, in connection with the way in which their organisations are structured and operate. To be involved in the process of management, or to be a manager in a government department or hospital perhaps, is often viewed – even today, some two decades on from the first major tranche of public sector reform – as something essentially different from perceived practice in the commercial sector. That there undoubtedly are differences is something that will be discussed later in this chapter. However, it must surely be as true for the public hospital administrator as it is for the insurance company executive that management is fundamentally about giving direction to an organisation, handling and anticipating problems and difficulties, and ensuring that organisational activity is in alignment with the expectations and needs of all customer groups. This is certainly the premise upon which this and subsequent discussion of IKM is based.

Information without knowledge: the road to IKM

It is a truth universally acknowledged, as Jane Austen might have said, that you can seek to manage information without necessarily setting out to manage knowledge. Indeed, there is much to be said in relation to the benefits that can accrue from adopting an incremental approach to implementing an IKM strategy as opposed to attempting to move to a fully integrated approach from the outset.

To consider first the term 'information society': it has been with us now for over a decade, stemming largely from the proliferation of data generation, storage and manipulation opportunities afforded by the development of ICTs and the impact that they have had upon the way we live. The fundamental contribution of these technologies has been to enable the gathering and storage of much more data about people, activities and processes than has ever previously been possible. Yet much of what has been captured has been data without purpose: statistical information, personal information that is gathered and retained because it is held to be enough justification that it is possible to do so. Often, such data are capable, upon interpretation and management, of being translated into information, something that has both meaning and possible application and consequent value. In order for this transformation to take place, however, there is a need for information parameters and procedures to be explicitly delineated and, where appropriate, for systems and software applications to be utilised to ensure that relevant data is integrated and organised to achieve the maximisation of appropriate use and relevance. In essence, what we are seeking to do is to create a soil and climate in which both information and knowledge management strategies can flourish. Such an environment cannot be bought from a packet off the shelf; rather, it requires careful husbandry and an acknowledgement, as we have already stressed, that the essential climate for knowledge management to grow and succeed is one where information management has already prepared the ground.

The process of managing data with a view to transforming it into information is a complex strategic one, which should be informed by an understanding of the way in which the organisation itself works. The role of information management, and by association the information manager (although, importantly, the job title itself can vary enormously and in many instances does not yet exist at all), is to determine what can most usefully and 'profitably' be gained from interpreting data which, upon human interface, takes on some meaning or application, either in isolation or in combination. The essential identifier of data to information transformation is the assignment of some meaning that is capable of human interpretation.

While theoretically complex, it becomes somewhat easier to understand the logic underpinning this process when it is considered in an applied context. For example, in many countries national or regional governments register motor vehicles on an annual basis. The data that is submitted by individuals is, in itself, often of limited value: it gives details of vehicle manufacturer and model, and the registration address, all primarily of importance in matters of vehicle-associated crime. However, by setting carefully constructed parameters, it is possible, from the mass of data collected regionally or nationally, to extrapolate information that is of greater value: of value to the 'owning' department, certainly, but capable too, within an integrated system, of producing supporting information for other departments within the same overarching administration. Indeed, it may possibly extend beyond this and be of value to external organisations. This concept of making use of opportunities afforded by the information-gathering

interaction has led some areas of the United States to use vehicle registration processes as an opportunity to encourage citizens to register for local
and national elections.

Yet this transformation does not take place miraculously. As yet, even the
most sophisticated software products can do no more in their own right
than identify trends emerging from data. The parameters for the creation of
information from data remain reliant upon the human interface, which is
perhaps why the quality and usefulness of the information that is generated
are often somewhat variable. As we shall explore in Chapter 2, there is a very
real need for an overarching organisational information strategy to give both
a foundation and a coherence to the task of extracting, using and managing
information.

Knowledge management and its relationship to information management

It is somewhat ironic that although in the late 1990s the terms 'knowledge
management' and the 'knowledge economy' entered the favoured lexicon of
senior managers for the first time (KPMG 1998b), for many of them it was
without any sense of how their organisations actually managed their information holdings. Without wishing to be overly simplistic, it is probably true
to say that sufficient and appropriate 'information' was deemed to exist
because supporting technologies had been put in place over a period of
years and had continued to develop in their processing power and sophistication, and that these information holdings and processes were largely
considered to be unrelated to the achievement of knowledge management.
Knowledge, on the other hand, was, when identified as a concept, usually
seen as something separate, removed from the information acquisition and
interpretation processes, requiring careful consideration and investment in
staff development, as well as in still more sophisticated computer software
packages.

Against the misleading assumption that information management is
something that can largely be left to ICTs and associated specialists to
achieve, the reverse has largely been true for knowledge management. There
has been almost uniform acknowledgement that there is a need to achieve
significant cultural change to persuade people of the value of sharing their
accumulated experiences and ideas with one another, and here the technology has taken on the supporting role that we have alluded to throughout
this chapter. 'The music is not in the notes,' observed the composer Charles
Ives, 'it is in the musician.' Human intelligence represents too complex, too
inherently unsystematic an asset base to ever be more than supported
through the deployment of ICTs (Angel 1998: 23).

However, what should be apparent already, particularly in the light of
the model of IKM represented in Figure 1.1, is that just as data is the raw

material from which information can be generated, knowledge is the product of information having been considered, perhaps applied, and reviewed. Without good access to appropriate information in the right format, available at the right time and accessible to the right people, the knowledge generation and sharing processes are likely to be considerably diminished in value. Thus, if there is to be any universal 'truth' emanating at this early stage, it is that a properly formulated strategy for information management without an explicit focus on knowledge management is likely to deliver far more, in respect of beneficial outcomes, than a knowledge management initiative undertaken in a vacuum, where information management is not prioritised in a clearly focused manner.

So knowledge management is not where organisations should be targeting all of their interest and resources. Rather, it is something which should be seen as being a natural progression from the foundations of good information management practice. Focusing on the nature of data to information transformation in a way which is reflective of the needs of the organisation should be the first key area of concern and activity. By doing this, and putting in place a framework where information is routinely shared and built into the decision-making processes, the first steps towards the creation of a knowledge-based and, ultimately, 'learning' organisation are taken. Thus, in the course of this text, it is the management of information which provides the foundations for the first chapters, from which we move naturally to consider ways in which knowledge management can be developed. It is only in the concluding section that we begin to consider what IKM can be when all aspects of the process are integrated into what is, for almost all organisations, an essentially new way of working; considering what it means to manage information and knowledge cannot help but impact upon what your organisation actually looks like.

'But we are different ...': managing information and knowledge in the public sector

Those of us who did not develop an interest or participate in the delivery of public services before the advent of what have become universally known as the linked periods of 'Reaganism' (1980–88) and 'Thatcherism' (1979–90) have grown up within a culture that views the terms 'bureaucracy' and 'government' as problems in search of a cure rather than models of service delivery with underpinning rationale. Among the twenty-first century railings against 'big government', there is a danger that we neglect the fact that this model of public service delivery was lauded, relatively few decades ago, as the way forward for post-war development, advocating a model that has been applied globally; as Weber asserts:

The decisive reason for the advance of bureaucratic organizations has always been its purely technical superiority over any other form of organization ... Precision, speed, unambiguity ... reduction of friction and of material and personal costs – these are raised to the optimum point in the strictly bureaucratic administration.

(Gerth and Wright-Mills 1958: 214)

So we see that the underpinning legacy of bureaucracy, often now disparaged, was once held up as a model of organisational effectiveness. The failures attached to it by Margaret Thatcher and her acolytes in North America and sections of Europe – and in the southern hemisphere led primarily by politicians in New Zealand and Australia – resulted, we are encouraged to believe, in radical dismantling of the bureaucratic structures that were dismissed as ineffective and wasteful methods for delivering public services. This philosophy of change is one that has also permeated former Eastern bloc countries where, since the collapse of communism, arguably the ultimate bureaucratic model, newly 'democratised' nations have been wrestling with the challenges of reforming and rebuilding the very fabric of their societies, following the complex and competitive model of 'democratic' governance.

Therefore the decades of the 1980s and 1990s were characterised by the sense of ongoing change that permeated organisations in the commercial sector, and the gradual encroachment of this culture into what can loosely be termed the 'public sector'. However, this very term is in itself problematic, for there is no neat, precise, globally applicable definition of what falls within the remit of the 'public sector'. For the purposes of this text, it is used to describe those services which governments, whether national, regional or local, provide, either directly or indirectly, to and for citizens (for example, these could include health care, education, social security and welfare services, defence, law and order, transport) and the supporting processes that governments must undertake in order to function effectively (revenue collection and legislation, to name but two). The sense of these public services and functions as being somehow 'different' from the commercial sector was one that was, superficially at least, challenged in the 1980s. The culture of change, driven by an increasingly competitive and globalising market, had begun to revolutionise manufacturing and private sector service industries in the 1980s; in many instances these were put forward as models of good practice which, if they could not be directly adopted, could at least be adapted for public sector deployment. However, too often change strategies applied across public services were compromised by a failure to acknowledge one key difference between the public and private sectors: 'Government and business are fundamentally different institutions. Business leaders are driven by the profit motive; government leaders are driven by the desire to get reelected' (Osborne and Gaebler 1992: 20).

Such a view is helpful at the outset in reminding us that we must be realistic about our study of the way in which the public sector can most usefully approach the management of information and knowledge. It is certainly true that, just as in the commercial sector, a sound business case has to be made for the adoption of IKM strategies, but for those operating in the public service arena there is a further dimension that complicates any move towards operationalising the management of either information or knowledge: there must be some 'political' payback associated with the changes and investment made. Public sector employees, although often and usually erroneously poorly regarded in respect of their management abilities and particularly their ability to facilitate and work with changing structures and models of service delivery, face challenges that their commercial sector counterparts do not: not only do they have to make and deliver a 'business' case, but they also have to be sensitive to the often shifting agendas of their political masters. In later chapters, when we consider particular aspects of IKM in relation to applied contexts, we should remind ourselves that critical success factors and, perhaps just as importantly, reasons for failure are, in the public service scenario, arguably more challenging and complex than their counterparts in the commercial sector. This is not a factor that is cited to excuse failure, but rather an acknowledgement that there is some excellent practice emerging from the public sector, a key tenet of which is represented by the way in which public service employees have learned from the commercial sector and have then risen to the challenge of tailor-making services and methods of service delivery which reflect the key political drivers with which they must work

So managing information and knowledge in the public sector is different, but as we shall discuss, perhaps not *that* different. The goals of creating organisations which fully utilise and value their information assets, and leverage the full potential of their people by tapping into formal and informal knowledge networks, should be common to organisations across the sectoral spectrum. However, for the public sector, there are additional challenges to be managed. Some, as we have already alluded, are fundamental to the nature of the political process itself, yet others, particularly in respect of legal and ethical constraints, are magnified many times over from those of the majority of their commercial sector counterparts. So perhaps, in respect of the management of information and knowledge, we would be better advised to acknowledge at the outset that it is the *difficulty* and *complexity* of the undertaking that represents the greatest challenge, instead of dwelling upon differences that may exist with practice in other sectors.

The road from 'one size fits all' to 'citizen-centric' public services

Having argued that the design and delivery of public services represents some unique challenges that are not mirrored in other sectors of the global economy, we must also acknowledge that the beginning of the twenty-first century finds public services facing a period of re-evaluation probably more fundamental than anything that was witnessed in the 1980s and 1990s. With the exception of China, which continues to pursue what can best be described as 'entrepreneurial communism', democracy, although variously interpreted, is the dominant model of public governance extant in the world today. A composite of various dictionary definitions of the term 'democracy' leads one to conclude that the foundation of the democratic process is the concept of 'government by the people'. Of course, such a definition steers one towards a pivotal assumption, which is that citizens intrinsically should have some interest in participating in the process of democratic government. However, there is little doubt that there is a growing trend towards a palpable and ingrained cynicism regarding politicians and the policies that they enact: for example, in historic bastions of the democratic process such as the United Kingdom and the United States of America, the level of dissatisfaction and resulting non-participation in the election process has led many commentators to conclude wryly that we get both the politicians and the services that we deserve.

Perhaps because of a realisation of the level of public dissatisfaction with politics and, by inference, the business of government, 'joined-up government' has become the battle cry of many senior politicians in Europe and North America since the late 1990s. A media soundbite certainly, but the concept of 'joined-up' thinking for reinventing the way in which government structures itself to do business and provide services offers the most significant opportunity for the linked disciplines of information and knowledge to make a significant contribution to the development of citizen-centric, efficient, effective models of public sector operations. 'Big government' – remote and complex government – has disenchanted those whom it exists to serve; it is resource-intensive at a time when almost all governments are seeking to keep their public spending in check.

So what will the future look like? Upton and Swinden leave us in no doubt that the not so very distant future will see us entering a period of 'information age government', where the generally held democratic principle of working for the good of society will be replaced by the citizen wishing to know 'what is in it for me?' (Upton and Swinden 1998). What will characterise the way that 'information age government' is structured, and what will make it different from the present models that we have worked with for at least the last two decades, and in many cases much longer than that? Again, Upton and Swinden argue that a move towards 'joined-up government', 'citizen-centric' government, or whatever you may call it, will be dependent upon five critical success factors. These are worth considering in some detail. In the first instance, they argue that a key aim must be to strive towards the integration of services:

Government services need to be integrated around customers' needs. There are a number of ways this can be achieved. For example, by life episodes (e.g. moving house or becoming unemployed) or around communities of interest (e.g. the elderly, immigrants, or the disabled). Private sector involvement will be essential in this process. This refocusing has enormous implications for how public service organisations structure themselves and their information systems. In addition, it will require changes in culture, for example shifting from a system in which staff are encouraged to stick to rules to one whereby they actively seek results; and new approaches to staffing and training. Increasingly, for example, there will be a need for multi-disciplinary staff, who can guide the public through the complexities of government services.

(Upton and Swinden 1998: 27)

Essentially, what is being referred to here is the need for government to enable itself to facilitate services in a more targeted and user-friendly manner. It will do this through the effective use and sharing of its information assets, whether by doing away with many departmental operating boundaries or by ensuring that public services are able to interact with one another in ways that render the service delivered both *meaningful* and *appropriate* to the customer. The role of the public sector employee as the enabler of access to these integrated services must surely be dependent for its success upon access, not only to appropriate information but also to the knowledge resources that underpin the successful delivery of these 'joined-up' ways of working.

The second of the critical success factors identified focuses upon the imperative to build partnerships across public services as well as with external agencies:

Providing well integrated services will require building relationships with government departments, libraries, police forces and health and voluntary agencies, as well as with the private sector, including banks, post offices, supermarkets and the more traditional suppliers into the public sector. This could be achieved through the use of private finance, joint venture companies, or local authorities being responsible for all citizen-facing services once the appropriate legislation is put in place.

(Upton and Swinden 1998: 27)

Although some of the terminology used in this argument for building partnerships suggests a provenance that roots it within the context of United Kingdom applications, the underpinning theme is of global significance. We know that such partnerships already exist to a greater or lesser extent in many countries. However, not yet having been fully explored – and of central importance to the way in which partnership relationships actually work in practice – are the parameters within which information and knowledge assets are managed to take account of the benefits that may accrue from opening up and sharing access to such resources, and the related issues of information security and the protection from commercial and other forms of exploitation of personal or politically sensitive information and knowledge assets.

Upton and Swinden are advocates of the 'local' approach to public service delivery, believing that the only way to overcome high levels of citizen disenchantment with the way in which the political system operates is to counter the remote and fragmented model of public service delivery with one which is truly integrated, utilising the most local level of service delivery to act as the public interface with all levels of government service. To do this effectively, they argue, there is an imperative at the outset of the re-engineering of these services to consult with your citizens:

> Local authorities need to find new ways to consult with their citizens on how services should be delivered. This could be achieved through citizens panels and juries, opinion polls, referenda or age-interest forums facilitated by IT. Feedback from these into the corporate strategy is essential. Technology has a major part to play in consulting the community. Paper-based questionnaires or telephone surveys can be long winded and it takes time to disseminate the results back to citizens. For example, email, video conferencing and public information kiosks could make this process immediate.
>
> It is important to remember, however, that training is essential for some of these, to enable citizens to choose their own issues. Providing an easy access to services and encouraging citizens to participate in shaping service delivery will have enormous impact on the democratic process.
>
> (Upton and Swinden 1998: 27)

If there is perhaps one caveat that should be recorded with regard to this particular view of the importance of citizen consultation, it is that in many instances the value of what is collected during these processes is perhaps of somewhat questionable importance. This is not to deny the importance of giving citizens a sense of involvement in, and ability to comment upon, the services provided and their levels of satisfaction with them: the sense of ownership, interest in and willingness to participate in the democratic process is absolutely essential if the democratic model of governance is to continue to grow and develop globally. However, whether the greater proportion of citizens are in a sufficiently well-informed position to make more than superficial input to the restructuring of public services is questionable.

An analogy drawn from previous research is helpful in contextualising this statement: in the design of motor vehicles, the input from existing customers, sought because in terms of public relations it is perceived to be a 'good thing' to be seen to consult your customer groups, in reality has little impact upon new product development. The reason for this lack of impact is explained by the limitations placed upon the individual's ability to imagine key facets of a new product through their accumulation of personal experiences of current and older models. As for motor vehicles, so too for public services: we know perhaps what citizens do not like, and this is important; we may be able also to ascertain what they perceive to be a well-structured service, drawn from the other sectors with which they interact. But as for the citizen being well placed to recommend a new architecture of public service delivery: this, it must be said, is questionable and leaves open the challenge for key strategists to map a future model of service delivery, in which the role of the information and knowledge manager(s) may well be pivotal (Milner 1997a: 121).

Access to services is the fourth of the key tenets put forward as being central to the achievement of 'information age government':

> Technology has an enormous role to play in ensuring that citizens have even access to all services. It makes it possible to deliver services into the home, workplace, or in a public place by phone, computer or face to face. The technologies needed to achieve this are here today: the Internet and Intranets, call centres, communications infrastructures that allow voice, data and pictures to be sent over the same cabling, plus mobile phones, faxes, PCs and interactive TV.
>
> (Upton and Swinden 1998: 27)

As has previously been briefly discussed in this introduction, and will be more fully developed in Chapter 4, the potential of information and communications technologies for impacting beneficially upon the delivery of public services is immense. Unfortunately, commensurate with the potential benefits are the opportunities, apparently all too frequently seized upon, for enacting poor decision-making in respect of information and communications technologies strategies. It is perhaps an overly simplistic view, but it bears close examination that the public sector has been extremely good at seizing the perceived opportunities afforded by investment in technologies, while unfortunately at the same time paying insufficient attention to the information and communications capabilities of what they have purchased. Once more, from the aspiration of achieving 'information age government', we can see that concealed just beneath the surface is a need to have, as a minimum, an understanding of the information and communication processes that exist across functions and operations.

The fifth and final critical component of Upton and Swinden's view of a reengineered and refocused public sector is characterised by what they refer to as the 'transfer of resources':

> By integrating services and sharing resources with each other, government departments and agencies, local authorities and community bodies can cut down on administrative duplication, for example home visits for first time benefit claimants or assessment of the elderly. Also by introducing call centres, public information kiosks and one-stop shops, citizens can adopt a more 'self-service' approach to their enquiries and transactions thus reducing the number of telephone calls, letters or visits handled by government offices.
>
> This will free up precious resources for local authorities and government departments, allowing them to focus on quality and the development of new citizen-focused services.
>
> (Upton and Swinden 1998: 27)

Reducing waste by impacting upon the amount of duplication that takes place is, as we discussed earlier in this chapter, one of the key goals of those seeking to manage information and knowledge. The argument, of course, is that by utilising resources in a more efficient manner (primarily by ensuring that access to such sources is available in the right place, at the right time and in the appropriate format), information age government can move from a position of largely being rhetorical to one of applied reality.

IKM – difficult, but not impossible

Throughout this chapter there has been an emphasis upon the challenge that is represented by attempts to identify, structure and manage information and knowledge assets, and it is right that this should have been so, for these are inherently complex processes. We have stressed, too, the common misconceptions that arise, particularly when discussing the management of information and its relationship to information and communications technologies. The task in subsequent chapters is to bring into focus, through exploration of both the theoretical and the applied, what it actually means to manage information and knowledge; and critically to focus on the way in which public sector organisations must structure themselves to do business in an operating environment that is increasingly the subject of review and reform by politicians.

The all-pervasive nature of both information and knowledge processes helps to define and problematise the very complexity of the task that we are addressing here. To create an environment where not only thinking but processes, too, are integrated, requires considerable and considered review of the way in which the diverse body of organisations making up the modern interpretation of the 'public sector' both generate and use information and knowledge. It is only by moving to a position of understanding what it means to treat information and knowledge as assets of considerable value, particularly in respect of their potential impact upon leveraging the efficacy of work carried out on behalf of citizens, that IKM can begin to replicate, in a public sector context, some of the powerful deliverables that commercial sector organisations are increasingly attributing to it.

The task, then, in subsequent chapters, is to move to establish an applied framework for managing information and knowledge while acknowledging and addressing some of the very considerable concerns that arise from it, particularly those impacting upon organisations within the public sector with regard to issues of freedom of information, data protection and the exacerbation of social exclusion. As we move forward from this introductory position, the feeling should be one of undertaking a journey through largely uncharted territory: it is certainly daunting, but not impossible. The final destination, indeed the core of the hypothesis underpinning this work, is one where managing information and knowledge demonstrate a capability to have a profound and ultimately beneficial effect on the operation of services undertaken on behalf of citizens by their governments, and on increasing opportunities for achieving effective and meaningful end-user engagement with, and involvement in, informing the development of models of public service delivery.

Chapter 2

Developing an information policy and strategy

The foundations of information management

The formulation of organisational policies and strategies should serve as a road map for both the short- and medium-term development of structures and practices. Thus, the development of an overarching policy in the area of information management should be seen as critical in providing the rationale and operational direction for the appropriate emergence of strategies for deployment of IM tools and techniques. In the public sector, there are increasingly examples of policy development activity in this area. Encouragingly, the development of such policies and subsequent strategies is clearly demonstrating an emerging awareness of the importance assigned to managing the information itself, as opposed to focusing almost in totality on the role of the associated technologies. This is a view developed by Strassman, who argues that:

> To manage information successfully, policy makers must set forth explicit principles for information governance and secure cooperation … Full disclosure of the rules for governing must indicate who will deliver what results and how the policy will be enforced. Therefore, policy pronouncements should be made only after allowing for adequate time and consideration, especially if they publicize the rules of information governance.
>
> (Strassman 1995: 5–6)

When analysing the key components of Strassman's account of the essentials of policy development, we are left to reflect on the importance of what he refers to as issues of 'governance' (Strassman 1995: 5). If properly developed, these may be said to provide the framework for IM and through implementation, as we shall discover later, to act as key supporting instruments in the achievement of KM.

Formulating an information policy: words are cheap?

Developing an information policy for public sector organisations, indeed for any organisation, is a complex undertaking: complex for many reasons, but inherently more difficult than areas such as financial or human resource management, due to the very fact that such resources, beyond issues of data protection and in some instances freedom of information, are traditionally poorly regulated and only rarely reviewed through external gatekeepers such as auditors or trade unions. During the course of this chapter we will review a high-level, overarching information policy, that of the Australian Commonwealth Government which sets out principles of IM for a major global economy and nation-state, serving to illustrate useful first steps in articulating public sector policy objectives in this area.

In considering this Australian example, encouraging as it is, a further set of issues will undoubtedly emerge, primarily around the way in which such policies can actually be implemented and, critically, the strategic processes that need to come into play if they are to have real operational impact. It is perhaps too easy to be cynical when discussing matters around policy development when, of course, what most of us are interested in are the end results balanced against any associated costs. However, for all areas of management the policy formulation stage represents the opportunity to gather views, to look at existing practice and to marry these against the agendas of those who control the organisations: senior managers, of course, but fundamentally, in the public sector, the views of political masters provide a further policy imperative that must be addressed.

An IM policy checklist

Developing policy in any sector is a complex and often time-consuming exercise. In order to be successful, there is a need to consider the way in which the organisation is structured internally and how it operates and is perceived externally, and to look at comparable policy development in other organisations. When focusing specifically on information management, there are a number of questions and issues that should be addressed at the outset. Taken together, these form an underpinning structure for some of the key issues that an information policy should address and galvanise a series of actions which, through appropriate strategy development, can ensure that 'worthy words' in policy documents are translated into tangible organisational improvement.

At the outset of policy development activity, there is a need in the IM area to ask a number of fundamental (and perhaps, at first sight, overly simplistic) questions which, when properly addressed, are capable of providing insight into the current organisational position as well as acting as indicators of the hoped-for eventual destination:

• Who is taking the lead in the development of an IM policy? What, if any, other areas of responsibility do they hold within the organisation?

- Does the organisation already have policy, strategy or guidance documents that contain the word 'information' in their title? If so, then they need to be looked at, in respect of both their provenance and the degree to which they have been actioned.
- What, if any, legislation, regulations or structures currently govern the flows of information across the organisation?
- Do any persons or job specifications, training or appraisal programmes in the organisation actually refer to IM as being something that is required of, or developed in, personnel at various operating levels?
- What does the organisation wish to gain from the development and deployment of an IM policy?

Undoubtedly these are critical questions that should be asked at the outset of any policy-development exercise, but the scale of the task represented here should not be underestimated. To ask and even attempt to answer these questions for a national government, as, say, in the case of Australia, represents a huge and potentially time-consuming undertaking, which in order to succeed requires one critical thing: *that the leader of the IM policy development activity has the mandate and authority to both ask and receive required answers to the questions outlined above.*

The critical issue of providing thought leadership and authority to both policy development and implementation activity is one that has been championed through the valuable work of the IMPACT programme. Although primarily addressing its work to those in the commercial sector, this has made a valuable statement, highly pertinent to those operating in the public sector, with regard to the need for senior level responsibility for issues in this area to be accepted and assigned:

> The Board of Directors is responsible for the assets of the organisation it governs and those assets owned by others to which it has rightful access; information is an increasingly vital asset in most organisations and is subject to changing risks and opportunities. It is an asset that is less well understood and less well handled than other recognised assets (e.g. property, financial assets). Given the immaturity of practice in this area and the potential risks and opportunities ... the Board should take a systematic approach to ensure appropriate policies and practices are in place and to check the adequacy of their arrangements for information assets.
>
> (IMPACT Ltd 1994: 7)

In place of 'Board of Directors', in the public sector we will often be substituting senior public service terminology, but the message remains the same: information management is a serious organisational issue and opportunity and, as such, it requires that very senior managers are identified with it in respect of both developmental and operational matters.

The IMPACT programme further identified a number of areas where it felt that policy development work should be prioritised, and with two important additions these provide an architecture for what a framework for action in respect of IM might look like:

• the classification of information assets;
• the quality of information provided;
• the proper authorised use of information for its rightful purpose;
• the identification of risks and appropriate protection;
• maintenance and exploitation;
• the development and implementation of information systems strategies.

(IMPACT Ltd 1994: 7)

and additionally:

• the relationship of IM to other areas of organisational activity;
• the identification and clarification of roles and responsibilities in respect of IM.

Each of these criteria merits closer examination in respect of policy development activity. Let us consider first the important issue of *classification* of information. Such a term has two distinct but important strands to its definition. The first relates to the information as an 'object' or 'item' itself and how that may be best organised for use. Imagine a scenario, across a complex but necessarily large operating structure, where over time a culture has been permitted to develop whereby essentially identical information processes and systems use entirely different vocabularies, and sometimes structures, to achieve fundamentally the same outcomes. Plot – or at least attempt to – your way through this confusing mix of terminology and you are likely to end up at best frustrated, at worst confused, and in both cases will probably achieve only a partial picture of what is available. By recommending the adoption of common thesauri, a controlled operating language, across organisations, you are building towards an information culture which is focused upon maximisation of use and minimisation of confusion in matters relating to all information-based functions.

A working example of this immense potential for confusion and waste to occur was observed in a higher education institution. This was organised into four distinct operating units for the delivery of academic programmes, but channelled the majority of its administrative and support activities through centralised units, as many such organisations do. In theory this should not in itself represent a significant IM problem with regard to 'classification'; however, the practical operational reality was somewhat different, for in the four 'academic' units observed, each used different terminology to describe what was essentially identical practice. The result, which can be seen in many similar organisations, was often confusion, inaccuracy and delay, all common and 'costly' outcomes of poor IM.

A second aspect of classification moves beyond the essentially structural issues outlined above, and relates to the concept of viewing information holdings as 'assets' to be both managed and used. The Hawley Committee Report, resulting from the work of the IMPACT programme, gives some useful pointers as to the way in which, in a public sector context, it should be possible to move towards some degree of classification on the basis of asset assessment:

> Classification of information assets is important in order for an organisation to identify those assets that merit special attention and to categorise them in terms of their treatment e.g., publicly available, internal, confidential, secret ... For the purposes of identifying and developing a shared understanding of the value of information assets for suitable classification, the main criteria that most organisations used were ... The impact on the organisation of theft, damage, loss, abuse or misuse of information ... Potential to increase revenue and reduce costs. Customer information was regularly identified as having potential, when integrated in particular ways, to generate revenues and reduce costs; for instance ... by more efficient handling of case-files giving significant reduction in costs.
>
> (IMPACT Ltd 1994: 8–9)

Classification as described, then, is essentially a dual-faceted process, both elements of which are clearly focused upon the achievement of organisations structured to perform better. The first area of focus relates, as we have said, to moving to a position where there is some logic underpinning the way in which information is generated and used; at its most fundamental, when information items exist, there must be a common and transparent methodology for identifying them, rather than the often muddled and confusing practice that currently exists in far too many organisations. Such a shift in practice links to the addition of value and maximisation of utility associated with what are often referred to as 'information assets'. Fundamentally it is the capability for improvement in performance, being able to identify and deploy, often through integration across a variety of operating 'boundaries', that best represents the critical need to focus on issues of information classification at the policy development stage.

In practice, issues of classification offer the best opportunity to achieve positive outcomes early in the life cycle of policy deployment. A move to common thesauri, while deceptively simple, does help to ensure that organisational information assets take on a coherence in use, which should serve to minimise both confusion and resulting time-wasting. Developing and main-taining a common operating language, however, is a challenge that should not be underestimated, particularly if the goal of the information policy is to facilitate information sharing and use across a complex public sector structure. An example of the scale of the undertaking represented was observed in the operating structures of a regional government on mainland Europe serving a population of some two million people; here, within six distinct functional units ranging across such areas as transport services and local taxation, there were found to exist seven separate terms used to 'clas-sify' one single entity, the individual external end-user. Even in this one simple example, the potential for confusion and time-wasting when analysing use and satisfaction is immediately apparent when one considers that no single manager or senior team appeared either aware or indeed concerned that those in their operating constituency were variously termed 'clients', 'patrons', 'customers', 'citizens', 'users', 'items' and, perhaps best of all, 'UoAs' – an abbreviation of 'units of activity'!

Now while it is true to say that, as end-users of public services, most of us actually care little how such organisations describe us, the potential impact of moving to a common operating language should not be underestimated. Increasingly there is an acknowledgement that public sector organisations should be capable of operating in a much more inter-disciplinary and cross-functional manner; this is not only resource-efficient but also brings with it the associated potential for leveraging the end-user experience of interaction with such services. However, the impact of good IM practice on the achieve-ment of such a mode of delivery must be realised. To some extent it is possible to argue that for work on the development of concepts of informa-tion classification to have real impact, such initiatives need to be undertaken at the most viable macro level – therefore, an example within regional government might be that it is desirable for all such structures to work towards the adoption of a common thesaurus, one which is monitored and maintained co-operatively and which is transparent for use by other agen-cies, be they central government or the voluntary or private sectors. Such a means of classification, or controlled language as it is sometimes called, is capable of ready access, maintenance and deployment through the harnessing of technologies such as Intranets and database management systems.

Moving beyond the foundations of a controlled language approach to information classification, the further dimension, alluded to previously in this chapter, of working towards classification on the basis of 'asset value' represents an important stage on the road to developing an organisational culture that embeds good IM practice as a matter of routine. There are two key drivers which could be said to underpin the development of a public sector philosophy of identifying and managing information assets: the estab-lishment of criteria which allow for the assessment of both

> The impact on the organisation of theft, damage, loss, abuse or misuse of information. Examples of this are: critical operational information that, if lost, brings the organisation to a halt, or information that, if leaked, would seriously damage reputations.

and

> Potential to increase revenue and reduce costs. Customer information was regularly identified as having potential when integrated in particular ways and reduce costs; for instance ... by more efficient handling of case-files giving significant reduction in costs.
>
> (IMPACT Ltd 1994: 8–9)

By moving in the first instance to identifying areas of commonality across the organisation(s) in respect of information holdings, and deploying a controlled language for maximising their visibility and use, the analogous issues of asset valuation become immediately more transparent as awareness grows of what information is actually gathered, used and archived. Having attained this position, it is possible to put forward an expectation in a statement of policy that issues of risk, in respect of loss, damage or theft of certain types of information, can be more accurately predicted. Further, an increased awareness of what information is held across an organisation opens up the possibility and real potential for the identification and exploitation of linkages and synergies, which may beneficially impact on the way in which the organisation *works*.

At a policy level, then, what is critical in respect of the issue of classification is, first and most important, that it is visible and is given some degree of prominence from the outset. Further, responsibility and scope for developing the policy in this area need to be clearly delineated, with an indication of the anticipated time-scale for delivery and a statement of intent with regard to both monitoring progress and seeking to come into alignment with other modes of classification identified in related organisations.

Policy on the quality of information provided

The explosion in the deployment and use of information and communications technologies has brought about an exponential growth in the ability of organisations to gather and process data. However, there are significant issues arising from the actual quality of this data, its fitness for purpose and the way in which, through use, it becomes information. As Tozer argues:

> this huge growth in our capability for producing and our appetite for consuming information has not been accompanied by improvements in the quality of the data itself. What is not sufficiently addressed by any of

this marvellous technology is the inherent correctness, completeness, simplicity and fitness for purpose of the data itself. Although Information Technology has grown from the precious child of the Sixties to the equally remarkable adult of the Nineties, losing its innocence and gaining a lot of responsibility along the way, it has yet to come to terms with the consequences of one of its own early maxims. Even today, Garbage In still almost invariably results in Garbage Out.

(Tozer 1994: 4)

Within a policy statement on IM there is undoubtedly a need to prioritise, in close alignment with the issues of organisation and classification previously discussed, the critical importance of the inherent and consistent quality of the information generated, used, being understood and managed. Partial, inaccurate and late information are all potentially dangerous and costly outcomes of poor focus on information quality. To this end, a policy document should set out the requirement for clear protocols on the consistency and accuracy of information gathering and presentation and on the timeliness of delivery. It should also address itself to issues of access and responsibility for updating and deletion for, as a matter of good practice, rights and responsibilities need to be clearly assigned in respect of information holdings – just as they would in the area of financial management, for example. There is, too, an increasing need for issues of information quality to take account of the matter of information overload. As has been observed in recent years, the huge growth in email communication has brought with it associated costs in respect of too much information flowing to too many people, often inappropriately, causing frustration, time-wasting and overload of the technological base of the organisation.

To summarise, key concerns around matters of information quality that should be addressed through IM policy documents appropriate for organisations in the public sector, are likely to include reference to all of the following:

• issues around the quantity of information flowing around the organisation and tangible costs associated with these purposes, balanced against the demonstrable fitness for purpose of the information itself;
• the ease with which it can be accessed, measured against any security requirements that may pertain;
• the efficiency of information-gathering systems and appropriate methodologies for sharing, in particular highlighting the potential of good practice to reduce any duplication of effort or wasted time in accessing required items;
• the desirability of achieving consistency in respect of the quality of content, terminology used and style of presentation;

- in respect of information available electronically, a requirement that the technologies deployed should be fully compatible with one another;
- explicit statements of clear parameters relating to both authority and responsibility for entering and amending information, in order that the accuracy and validity of the information can, as far as possible, be guaranteed.

It is in this area of information quality that perhaps the most tangible operational issues of concern to IM pertain, and as we shall discuss in subsequent chapters, these are also of critical importance in underpinning the evolution of knowledge management. Contained within the checklist outlined above is a blueprint for action that can be couched in terms with which senior public sector managers should feel both familiar and comfortable, for this is the language of *responsibility*, *accountability*, *standards* and *measurement*.

The 'proper use' of information

Defining what is meant by 'proper use' in respect of IM concerns addressing issues around achieving conformity to existing and emerging legal and perhaps regulatory requirements, and moving to define organisation or sector standards and ethical guidelines in respect of the management of information. As we shall discuss in Chapter 7, important legislation exists globally with regard to both data protection, where a key focus is upon protecting the rights of the person(s) referred to in the information holdings, and freedom of information, where issues of access dominate, but as yet there has been much less focus on the development of sectoral standards for IM practice.

In respect of operating standards, the starting point must be to acknowledge that there are likely to be three identifiable, but not necessarily always separate, roles in the IM process. First is the *owner* or *guardian* of the information, the individual or group with ultimate legal and/or management responsibility for the operation of the organisation, who must bear ultimate responsibility for issues such as loss, theft or inaccuracy. The second of the linked roles is that of the *information keeper*, who at an operational level must ensure that information is generated, maintained, archived and deleted in an appropriate and, when necessary, secure manner, demonstrating full cognisance of legal and ethical directives emanating from the information owner. The final role in moving towards the achievement of proper use of information assets is that of the *user*. Here, too, rights and responsibilities must be clearly understood: rights in respect of the types and levels of information to which they may have access, and responsibilities in respect of what they can do with that information, once accessed – for example, do they have the right to amend, copy or delete information items?

A policy document cannot, in itself, go beyond stating in rather general terms the principles by which it intends that the organisation or sector should be structured to ensure 'proper use'. However, in moving to operationalising such policy, the issues of good practice, assignment of responsibility and monitoring of adherence, in both use and safekeeping, take on particular resonance when what is being managed is information relating to public services. A key determinant in commercial sector adoption of standards surrounding the use of information has generally been to maintain and leverage competitive position, an important and sensitive issue in itself. However, when the information item in question relates to the health or police record, benefits or taxation information relating to the private citizen, then these sensitivities and the potential for calamity are magnified many times over. This points us unquestionably to the need for statements of policy to be backed up by a widespread and significant investment in training the workforce. We must ensure that they have the information-handling skills and information 'sensitivity' appropriate to their role in the organisation, and that such programmes of training are regularly reviewed and updated in alignment with developments in information management practice within the organisation.

On issues of proper use, there is an additional area of concern that should be addressed at the highest levels: the need to acknowledge that the responsibilities of good practice pertain not only to internally generated and 'owned' information. Certainly, the greatest focus in IM is upon those assets which can be identified as belonging in some way to the organisation. However, there are considerable pitfalls associated with the failure to acknowledge that organisations have responsibility for good management practice, as well as possible legal requirements in respect of information that is generated externally and acquired for use within the organisation. Examples of such practice might involve breaching legal copyright by circulating copies of market intelligence reports beyond admissible numbers. Or, in matters of contract tendering, jeopardising the impartiality and reliability of the bidding process by failing to control access to tender documents. As the process of public governance becomes increasingly complex, with much more involvement and interaction with external agencies, the need for clear protocols to safeguard potentially sensitive information which is routinely exchanged must be considered a priority in moving towards a view of what is meant by 'proper use'.

Identifying and protecting information from risk factors

It is appropriate to consider issues of risk in close proximity to our discussion of the setting out of protocols for 'proper use'. Across public sector organisations there are, as yet, no clear and generalisable patterns of what can be said to represent 'risk' associated with the management of information. This is because the types of information held, and the relative value that they represent to the operation and security of the department, authority or agency in question, are likely to differ considerably. However, a helpful definition of some of the key considerations which should be taken into account when formulating a policy on information-related risk management has been put forward in the 1998 responses to an annual survey on the question of information security; here, 'information security is defined as practices and procedures which ensure that information, generally held in electronic format, is safeguarded from unauthorised access, modification or accidental change and is readily available to authorised users on request' (Information Security Survey 1998: 1).

While this definition is helpful in moving the issue of risk and security to the forefront of the IM agenda, what it does not explicitly state is the requirement for issues of risk and security to be classified as to the relative value of different information assets to the organisation, yet this is pivotal to the provision of a policy capable of being moved from document into action, This classification will undoubtedly differ across organisations: for example, in a national government policy statement, such as that of Australia which we consider later in this chapter, issues of risk can only be flagged as matters of general priority, with a caveat that there is a need for sectors or organisations which represent operating subsets to audit their information holdings and to move to a position of risk management in respect of a properly informed understanding of what actually exists. The Hawley Committee Report suggests that, having audited information processes and holdings, it is then desirable to classify risk on the basis of a matrix measuring variance against the following three categories of risk:

*   the impact of the risk on the performance of the organisation (i.e. if the risk scenario came to pass, what would the effect of the predicted outcomes be?);
*   the likelihood of an incident occurring;
*   contextual factors such as time (e.g. payment of pensions and other benefits), information recipient (e.g. a citizen requiring notification of tax liability), place (e.g. local or national sensitivities) or presentation format (e.g. web sites, paper-based forms, call centres). These issues of when, where and how need to be considered, as they may materially affect the impact and likelihood of the risks occurring and demand particular measures (e.g. contingency plans for benefits payment in the case of major system failure resulting in loss or damage to citizen records).

(Adapted from IMPACT Ltd 1994: 17)

Identifying risk is only one part of the IM equation. Putting in place strategies to protect the organisation from predicted outcomes is something that can only be undertaken with the benefit of having assessed the likely impact of the risk against the indices outlined above. Responses and measurements based upon these indicators enable a methodology for classifying both the likelihood and predicted impact of the risk as against the actual costs of mechanisms to minimise or protect against it actually occurring, and should be viewed as a critical IM strategy focus. In essence, this should be a relatively straightforward cost/benefit analysis, but it is one that can only be said to be credible if those undertaking it and making decisions based upon the classification of risk actually have a strong conceptual and applied understanding of the importance of information to the organisation.

In the closing years of the twentieth century an excellent example of risk management and associated protection strategies regarding information assets concerned the issues presented by the problem of achieving Year 2000 compliance. In many ways, and despite the considerable degree of confusion and even panic that ensued within public sector organisations globally, this arguably apocryphal 'time bomb' has ensured that politicians and senior managers have been left in no doubt of the huge reliance of almost every public sector function on the generation, use and storage of information, at levels from the most basic data through to the most complex economic models. At the time of writing it is possible to reflect that, although the 'doomsday' scenario predicted by many commentators did not come to pass, the fear of the 'millennium bug' did at least increase the awareness of politicians and senior managers to the dependence of society and organisations upon electronically stored and accessed information resources.

Exploitation of information assets

As with any organisational asset, information is, more often than not, of both use and value in its own right, and an IM policy document should in the first instance point to the need for this to be the case. However, increasingly across all organisations and sectors including (usually belatedly, it has to be said) the public sector, a view is permeating whereby it is considered desirable to leverage the performance of all available asset groups by considering opportunities for 'adding value', usually through the exploitation of synergies that may exist across a number of functions or operating units. In an IM context, this usually concerns opportunities arising from policies that point to the desirability of encouraging the sharing and exchange of information in appropriate instances; these may include helping to achieve desired outcomes, such as perhaps an increased range of service offered with a more straightforward end-user interface, or reduced levels of duplication of effort in information gathering or processing. Responding to this trend in calls for value-added approaches to be incorporated into public sector practice, the International Council for Information Technology in Government Administration put in place a research group to consider issues of information sharing both within and between different tiers of government (ICA 1997a). Although not putting forward conclusive policy statements, this comparatively early-stage research is pointing to the fact that 'security and privacy issues are the greatest impediment to information sharing' while perhaps conversely 'public readiness and encouragement seemed more common than public resistance' (ICA 1997a: 3).

Within this apparent context of end-user readiness to welcome developments in the provision of public services based upon exploitation of the ability to share information assets across traditional service boundaries, a number of benefits of interest to policy-makers are immediately evident:

- end-users should benefit from enhanced and simplified experience of interacting with public sector services;
- there should be a focus upon the benefits that may accrue from the ability to make better use of the information provided by end-users, ideally resulting in a fall-off in the amount of duplicated information gathered and processed by individual agencies;
- the overall efficacy of both planning and decision-making processes at macro and micro level may be enhanced by having the opportunity to consider provision and performance in respect of a greater awareness of the overall operating scenario.

A further important aspect of the concept of exploitation in the IM area is closely linked, in respect of policy development, to issues which relate to the management of knowledge assets: even in an organisation that does not yet feel itself ready or desirous of setting out specific KM policies, there should nonetheless be some statement with regard to the likely importance of managing and exploiting intellectual, or 'people', assets in particular. By this, we mean that in putting forward aspirations for a more information-sharing, end-user focused mode of public service delivery, considerable opportunities may arise from harnessing the knowledge, ideas and observations of all strata of the workforce, thus moving towards the design of new modes of service delivery; and for greatest benefits to be gained from these assets, there is a need for some formalised mechanism for gathering and analysing such potentially important resources.

Issues of information exploitation must also be set within a policy context, in terms of what it is considered desirable to achieve. It is never going to be enough simply to eulogise in a policy statement about the concepts of sharing and exchange as being a 'good thing'; in order for them to be moved into applied and meaningful strategies, there is a paramount need for a statement of policy to point towards *why* such concepts represent a sound proposition for public services and *what* tangible outcomes it is envisaged they will achieve.

Information systems as an aspect of IM policy

One of the major problems associated with the advancement of a 'business' case for focusing on information management as an area of operation warranting both policies and strategies is that, in very many instances, senior level decision-makers are likely to suggest when questioned that they do already focus upon the importance of IM. However, in reviewing policy statements and annual reports from organisations as diverse as hospitals and mining companies, what becomes apparent at a very early stage is that issues involving 'information' as a concept are almost always referred to in the context of the technology-based systems that have been deployed within the organisations to process information. In research carried out in 1996 at the University of North London, analysis of some two hundred organisational annual reports, drawn from all sectors of the global economy, failed to find a single example of an instance where information was referred to in a context other than that of the investment made in technology-driven systems (Milner 1997a).

So there is, in a sense, something of a dilemma to be addressed here. It is one which we alluded to in the introductory chapter of this book, and it is fundamentally one of educating and raising the awareness of senior policy-makers to the value of the information which their organisations both generate and hold, and to their responsibility as senior managers for ensuring that maximum value is extracted from such assets. Undoubtedly, the role of information systems is an important one in respect of IM, but it is essentially a subsidiary one, a supporting and enabling position – one which represents considerable investment, certainly, but investment that should be informed by an awareness of what the organisation needs to do in respect of its information assets.

So while information systems are undoubtedly an important element in the 'recipe' that contributes to the development of an effective policy, they are also a potentially dangerous component – dangerous in that the place of systems, and the level of importance attributed to them, can be prioritised to the extent that they actually become the drivers of information policy rather than the key enablers. When this happens, and such instances are all too prevalent in public services, what can often result is poor information management resulting from considerable investment in technologies.

'Joined-up' policy: IM and other aspects of public service management

The development of an IM policy should not be carried out in a vacuum that takes no account of other areas of activity. Because information is all-pervasive, it underpins almost every process that is carried out, and care should be taken in framing a policy document to ensure that clear signposts highlight the way in which IM relates to and supports other key operational and strategic areas. Thus, an IM policy should indicate explicitly how it relates to areas such as: human resource management; training and education; service delivery; financial management; and, indeed, the technological areas discussed above. For this to happen, and to be further developed into meaningful strategies capable of effective deployment, there is likely to be a need for some degree of significant cultural shift to take place whereby the organisation or service demonstrates an awareness of its own internal structures and priorities in a non-territorial and mature manner and where, increasingly, policy will need to be framed to demonstrate awareness of, and facilitate co-operation with, other agencies and departments.

Identifying and clarifying IM roles and responsibilities

Although information is certainly all-pervasive in public service organisations, responsibility for managing it remains a largely undefined matter. Having worked to produce a policy based upon at least some of the factors outlined in this chapter, success or failure will subsequently rest upon the degree to which ownership of, and ultimate responsibility for, this area is assimilated at the most senior level. To cast any policy document adrift without ongoing husbandry and monitoring is to invite failure; in an area where issues of both concept and operational priority are complex and where it is often impossible to quantify their ultimate value and importance by recognised and accepted methodologies, the dangers are magnified many times over.

Thus, from the outset, an IM policy must clearly articulate the roles and levels of IM responsibility that it envisages throughout the organisation, beginning at the very top with an articulation of the role of the senior manager responsible for IM and acknowledging that this is a major portfolio of work, not something which can be simply 'bolted-on' to a traditionally more 'substantive' role. From this point of identifying senior level responsibility, the policy statement should then point towards a structure which assigns both roles and responsibility at all points in the organisation. Policy statements which suggest that 'information management is the responsibility of all staff' – and there are certainly a number of examples of such phrasing in existence – fail to address the degree to which the individual has a responsibility for the information which they both use and generate. In practice, employees can only be held accountable for their behaviour in relation to information if they themselves are working from a clear basis of understanding the information protocols upon which their own particular role is delineated; further, they must have a view of what IM actually means within the organisation, based upon ongoing training and development programmes as well as performance appraisal mechanisms which are appropriate to the operationalisation of the IM policy.

IM policy in action: the example of the Australian Commonwealth Government

There is a tendency, when discussing aspects of IM policy development, to attribute certain of its elements to be nothing more than 'common sense', or simply the application of 'motherhood and apple pie'. However, in any organisation, developing an effective IM policy is in fact a complex and potentially time-consuming exercise, dependent upon effective and focused leadership to bring it to the point of implementation. In a public sector context, 'political' considerations of almost every type, often complex and interrelated operating structures and limited financial resources all combine to provide challenging policy development environments, often around issues beyond the scope of immediately apparent 'common sense.'

The example of the information policy developed by the Australian Commonwealth Government is set out in summary form below as a case study of emerging good practice for consideration by those involved in all tiers of public sector management. It demonstrates the importance of taking a macro-organisational, perhaps even societal, view of IM, and then developing this in appropriate micro-operating contexts by demonstrating linkages to specific operating functions within the 'public sector' (Australia, Information Management Steering Committee on Information Management in the Commonwealth Government 1997). It is as yet too soon to attempt a reliable qualitative assessment of the success or otherwise of this policy; what it serves to do, in the context of this chapter, is to provide a worked example of what a statement of policy could look like.

The extracts set out below are taken from the statement on the 'Management of Government Information as a National Strategic Resource', in particular from the summary document which prefaces the document. However, perusal of the full document, available online at the Australian Commonwealth Government's web site (http://www.fed.gov.au/publications), is strongly recommended, as it provides what is, in a global context, arguably the best example to date of developmental work in this key area.

Importantly, the report begins by setting out a vision of public service for the year 2000 and beyond, one in which the principles of IM are deemed to be capable of making a key input:

> Our goal is better government – better government through grasping the opportunities presented by new technologies, and more effective, less costly government through improved information management policies and practices. Our vision is for a government that uses its information fully, as a national strategic asset of government, business and the community; manages information for better policy development and the continuous improvement of services; shares information easily across agency boundaries; improves information flows to promote collaboration

across the public service and with other levels of government; and protects personal privacy and the public interest. We see information management as a principal agent for change in the Australian Public Service (APS) – a key factor in the continuous improvement process. Improved coordination and cross-agency collaboration in information management will enable the Government to meet its objectives – improved productivity and service delivery – while ensuring public confidence that government is in control of its information.

> (Australia, Information Management Steering
> Committee on Government 1997: 1)

If we reflect on the components of policy development in the IM area discussed in this chapter, it is possible to identify that even in this, the opening section of the Australian document, much alignment with the indicators of good practice is already evident. It is worth noting in particular that this statement on IM is explicitly set within a much wider context and overall aspiration, which is focused upon moving forward a major change and improvement agenda for all aspects of public service delivery. A further articulation of this is provided within a statement of 'reasons' as to why IM is being prioritised:

> In the last decade, the APS reform agenda has recognised some essential elements of business practice requiring specific attention. All have aimed at changing the way the Commonwealth Government conducts its business, bringing it closer to its clients. Responsiveness, flexibility, timeliness, accountability and continuous improvement are all aims that have been sought through human resources and financial management reforms in individual departments and agencies.
>
> There have been significant recent advances in information technology, including reduced costs of data communications and electronic storage, wide area interoperability via standard networking protocols, universal document creation through electronic word processing and publishing, and user-friendly graphic interfaces. With these advances in technology, a whole-of-government approach to managing information has become both feasible and necessary. This presents us with an opportunity to establish and maintain a better relationship between government, our clients and strategic partners.
>
> If there is the investment in the infrastructure required for effective public dissemination of information and cross-agency collaboration, the Commonwealth Government can begin to work as a single organisation to provide quicker, cheaper and better administration and delivery of services. Reforms can lead to information being shared as easily across the APS, and beyond, as within an agency. Within a legislative framework ensuring that issues of privacy, confidentiality, national security

and national interest are satisfactorily addressed, information management reform can lead to quality information collection, creation and
feedback from many organisations and individuals – necessary elements
of quality government.

Greater availability of information also allows citizens to become
more active participants in government – better informed and better
equipped to demand high standards of service. They will no longer be
forced to deal passively with bureaucratic systems and processes which
often appear designed to frustrate and delay rather than to help. The
gap between the users of public services and delivery agencies can be
narrowed. Improved collaboration in information management across
all layers of government can provide universal, cheaper and easier
access for citizens to government.

Government will be able to contribute to the commercial sector –
both in providing easier and more timely access to valuable information
collected at taxpayers' expense and in reducing the frustrations for business in dealing with regulations and policies fragmented across the
current structures of government. Effective cross-agency information
management also can mean more effective business, and beneficial
public–private sector partnerships ...

The Commonwealth Government now needs to seize the opportunities
provided by the convergence of the new information and communication technologies. The current environment provides significant
opportunities for the Commonwealth to move forward towards a whole-
of-government approach, while mindful that it will take some years of
sustained effort to transform policy into practice by all APS staff.

To unlock this potential, government needs to become smarter in its
approach to information management. Unnecessary duplication can be
avoided, and common standards can reduce transaction costs and difficulties. But this requires not just the technology, but also commitment
by managers and staff to make the necessary structural changes, both
within and across agency boundaries.
(Australia, Information Management Steering Committee on Information
            Management in the Commonwealth Government 1997: 3)

Critically, this important agenda-setting introductory section concludes
by stating with some force that if any of the improvements introduced in
association with IM are to be achieved, 'it will require political direction and
leadership at both government and agency levels. In our view, the information management reform agenda needs champions at the highest political
and bureaucratic levels' (ibid.: 4).

Interestingly, at the time that this policy document was prepared in 1997,
it was driven by what was then known as the Office of Government Information
Technology (OGIT), a functional area of the Commonwealth Government

located within the Department of Finance. In 1998, the remit of OGIT was merged with those of advertising and public communications and assimilated into the Department of the Prime Minister, arguably moving the issues of IM to the policy-generating centre of Australian government. Whether this change of location and assimilation of other key areas has longer-term implications for the achievement of the IM agenda outlined above it is too soon to say. In one sense, the movement of IM to the policy-making area controlled by the country's elected leader is an encouraging move and one that potentially sends out strong messages of intent to all tiers and agencies of government located within the country. Additionally, a move to make explicit the linkage between IM and government communications strategies is also potentially extremely helpful in respect of leveraging the impact of the synergies to be attained from treating the two issues, when appropriate, in concert. However, there are also considerable dangers inherent in potentially diluting the overall function and direction of IM policy and strategy development by merging it with another area, such as communications, which may attract more overt 'political' attention.

To conclude our review of the Australian Commonwealth Government statement on IM, it is helpful to consider two statements of principle which serve to summarise a posited agenda for future development and deployment. These two sets of 'principles' are set within a statement of possibility:

> The Committee believes that information management reforms can make a major contribution to the Government's plans for reduction in the size and costs of the Australian Public Service, while at the same time ensuring the continuing improvement of services to the public. Some capital investment in technology, reskilling and organisational and cultural change will be needed to make this happen. But the costs of not making such investments will prove greater over the medium term.
> (Information Management Steering Committee on Information Management in the Commonwealth Government 1997: 4)

So the business case for moving to adopt IM principles is clearly made, but what does this mean in practice? For the purposes of this example, two sets of principles are set out, representing an underpinning road map of actions to be worked towards if the overarching goals and benefits alluded to are to be realistically achieved. These 'principles' are divided into two groups: those which articulate good practice with respect to what are referred to as issues of 'information service', and those which deal explicitly with 'principles of information management'. If we consider the former, we can see that they go some way towards expressing almost a 'bill of rights and outline of responsibilities' in respect of information issues:

Access to publicly releasable government information is a fundamental

right of all citizens in a democratic society. Government information is
a national resource and subject to privacy and security legislation and
directives and other legitimate government and third party interests,
agencies shall ensure that the information they hold is visible and that
information of potential value to individuals, the private sector and
other agencies is accessible.

Personal information shall be accessible only in accordance with
statutory privacy principles. Agencies are custodians of their information. They are responsible for: managing it, storing it securely and
describing it so as to make it visible and, where appropriate, accessible;
making it available for evidential and historical purposes; and archiving
it in accordance with government policy and legislation.

Agencies shall take due care to ensure the quality, integrity, security
and authenticity of government information.

Agencies shall provide information in accordance with their charter
and Commonwealth legislation and directives, and shall make the
following information freely available, or at no more than the cost of
dissemination: directories of services and organisation; information
needed by the public and organisations to understand their entitlements
to government assistance and the requirements of government which affect
them; legislative information, including bills, acts, treaties, subordinate
information, legislative status information, parliamentary timetables and
Hansard records; press releases, speeches and other public information
released by ministers, their officers and holders of statutory offices; other
documents and publications which are important to public understanding
of government activities and the organisation of government, including
annual reports, corporate strategic plans and other public accountability-
type documents reports required to be submitted to Parliament; a
statement of the categories of documents maintained in the possession of
the Government and the means by which the public may obtain access;
and information about their powers affecting the public, and manuals
and other documents used in decision-making affecting the public.

Agencies shall not gain a competitive advantage in their business
activities through privileged access to publicly releasable information.

In general, information provided as a by-product of budget-funded
activities, or directly through those activities, shall be available at no
more than the cost of transfer.

In order to facilitate public access to government-held information
and available services, the government shall work with a diversity of
access providers, including libraries and the private sector, to ensure that
government information is available in local communities.

(Australia, Information Management Steering Committee on Information
Management in the Commonwealth Government 1997: 6)

Such statements of 'service principle' are important, for they serve to move the whole issue of IM out from what, in this particular example, is by necessity a macro-level policy statement to a position where it is clear that it impacts and interacts with all tiers of government service and modes of delivery. The focus also explicitly centres the 'citizen' as being an important consideration in any IM 'equation'; public sector organisations have a duty, as articulated here, to concentrate on achieving appropriate levels of citizen engagement with information generated by publicly funded and accountable bodies.

If the set of service principles can be said to have externalised issues of IM, then the second set of principles put forward relate much more closely to the internal challenges that need to be addressed in order for IM to prosper in a public sector context. Fundamentally, it is stated that:

> In developing systems for the organisation, transmission and transaction of information, agencies should start from the premise that, subject to privacy legislation, all information content will at some time be transferred across agency boundaries, and design access systems accordingly.
>
> IT systems for common functions should be shared across agencies, where appropriate, to reduce development, operating and maintenance costs.
>
> Commonwealth records in all formats should be captured in appropriate record-keeping systems.
>
> Agencies should design systems which will, as far as possible, facilitate information being entered into electronic form only once, then being reused in many different ways through standard interapplication interfaces.
>
> User interfaces to government systems should be designed to present a consistent look and feel to users; common guidelines on the presentation of commonly used Information and series should be adopted.
>
> Commonwealth agencies should seek to cooperate with appropriate State and local government agencies in the management of information.
> (Australia, Information Management Steering Committee on Information
>   Management in the Commonwealth Government 1997: 12)

Drawing the policy strands together

At the outset of this chapter, a view of policy development as providing an underpinning and indeed essential foundation of the achievement of successful IM was put forward. Discussion of key components of such policy statements and consideration of a worked example of an extant policy statement should leave one in no doubt that, for an IM policy to have any impact or achieve any lasting benefit, it must be framed in a way which moves it beyond a mere expression of 'worthy intent'. Information management is a serious organisational proposition, capable of moving forward a substantive change and improvement agenda such as those commonly associated with the design and delivery of public services. If, in practice, it is not treated at the policy-setting stage as a serious and important statement of intent, to be driven forward by key senior organisational figures, then it is likely always to deliver limited or even disappointing returns. To paraphrase Tozer's view on information quality, what all those championing the development of workable and effective IM policies in a public sector context must work to avoid is a situation whereby worthy words *in* will lead to no more than worthy words *out*; to allow this to happen is to consign IM to almost certain failure (Tozer 1994: 4).

Chapter 3

Information management strategy in action

Making a 'business' case

In the opening chapters we have focused upon defining what in both theory and practice is generally meant by the management of information, and on the development of policies and strategies that can move at least some applied aspects of IM to an operational position. However, there is a danger that, in print at least, all of this can seem deceptively straightforward: it is enough to say simply, 'IM is important' or perhaps even 'critical' to the achievement of organisational success, and, as if by magic, policies and strategies to deliver both improvements and innovations in this area will gain widespread acceptance. The gap between the rhetoric of theory, even where expressed as well-crafted policy and strategy documents, and the reality of achieving *action* is one that is all too prevalent in the public sector domain, where complex, often legacy-based structures, scarce funding and, on occasion, conflicting political agendas can all serve to ensure that change operates only at the margins of an established *modus operandi*.

In Chapter 2, the need for senior-level championing of IM was highlighted as essential if it is to stand any chance of moving to a position of achieving operational impact. What we must now focus upon is the reality of what it means to be an IM 'champion' in a public sector context: that is, someone who is capable of engaging interest and commitment – through the power of persuasion and negotiation, certainly, but subsequently through being sufficiently in command of the IM brief to ask and seek answers to a number of mission-critical questions:

- How does an IM strategy link to the achievement of wider public service objectives?
- What are the critical aspects of management which support IM?
- What are the critical success factors?
- What is the ideal, the vision, to which you aspire?

Embedded within these questions is a critical hierarchy of focus, where at the outset you must ask – and, perhaps just as importantly, be seen to be asking – how IM will contribute to the achievement of a wider public service improvement agenda. By doing this, you can work towards ensuring that IM is explicitly located within the parameters of current operations and future change strategies. Subsequently, then, there is a need to ask and answer questions in relation to where IM *fits* within the wider management context: is it, for example within a health service scenario, linked to the ICT function or to clinical audit, or perhaps, as we shall see as we move to consider issues of knowledge management, located within human resource functions? Good practice and sound theory, as we have previously discussed, should lead us to a considered view that IM interacts with almost every management function that might be found within a public sector scenario. However, when moving to a position of deployment or action, it may be wiser and potentially more beneficial in the longer term to build linkages more slowly, to demonstrate first, perhaps, that IM principles can bring about significant improvements when adopted in relation to a discrete area such as clinical audit or pensions payment, and from this to move towards building links with other aspects and areas of operation.

Knowing or anticipating what factors will have the greatest impact on success depends very much upon having some clear articulation of what it is that you are aspiring to achieve. The case study of the Australian Commonwealth Government cited in the previous chapter leaves one in no doubt from the outset that it expects IM to make a significant contribution to the achievement of a reconfigured public service, one which is more focused upon its core functions and is demonstrably capable of managing multi-tiered relationships, both with partner organisations and with the citizen as end-user. Too often in the public sector – and we may hypothesise that this is as a result of the absence of a clear profit over loss motive – the vision or aspiration towards which efforts should be focused is so soft-edged that it is hardly surprising that there is much scope for misinterpretation or even manipulation.

Let us consider a further Australian example of public sector change in the light of the four areas of focus that have been highlighted as requiring both attention and understanding from the senior-level champion. Although not explicitly stated, it is perhaps indicative of the spread of take-up and influence of an underpinning IM strategy cited previously, that of the Centrelink initiative. On its launch in September 1997, its Chief Executive Officer, Sue Vardon, described this initiative as 'the biggest structural re-arrangement of Commonwealth Public Service delivery in fifty years' (Vardon 1998: 4). Vardon continues by describing the scope and scale of the challenge for which she is the senior-level manager:

> Centrelink offers an integrated range of services to *all* Australians, whether retired, studying, looking for work or homeless; as well as families, people from non-English speaking backgrounds and people with disabilities. The sheer breadth and diversity of Centrelink's client base

has created special challenges – but it has also inspired Centrelink's guiding philosophy: personalising its services to customers' individual needs.

(Vardon 1998:4)

A cursory glance at the aspirations set out in this statement can leave one in no doubt that this is an ambitious and complex undertaking, dependent almost entirely for success upon the ability of the operating agency to access and share information that was previously the domain of free-standing government agencies and departments. It also implies, through reference to the concept of 'personalising' services, that the client has become the primary focus in both design and delivery of service protocols.

However, if we reflect upon the first of the four questions which were set out at the beginning of this chapter to examine how an IM strategy fits with wider public sector objectives, we can see that, in reality, tensions may be apparent from the outset in the context of Centrelink, and indeed of many less ambitious projects currently operating globally. Often, when IM and ICT strategies are being put forward to represent an agenda for positive organisational change, they are, irrespective of sector, 'sold' at senior level as being capable of delivering significant efficiency gains. Unfortunately but not altogether surprisingly, improvements in efficiency are all too readily seized upon by senior mangers as representing opportunities for reducing staffing costs. Thus, in the case of Centrelink, while the rhetoric and indeed the theory surrounding its creation were laudable, the reality, in political terms, was the requirement of politicians that the change should result in significantly reduced government expenditure: thus Centrelink has been given the challenge of delivering improved citizen services but with a reduced core budget and a reduction in total staffing over the period 1998/99 of some 25 per cent. An Australian national newspaper commenting upon this situation noted:

While the Community and Public Sector Unions may have been highly critical of Centrelink and the job cut-backs associated with its attempts to meet its efficiency dividend, the information-technology industry was all admiration. A senior US IT executive assured us … that what Centrelink was attempting to do was right at the cutting edge and, if it worked, would be cited as a shining example of how other Governments should act. He did acknowledge, however, that the Centrelink strategy was technically complex and that it would be no easy task to get it up and running. Australia, it seems, is running much faster than most in pushing IT as an answer to Government service delivery.

(*Sunday Times* 1998: 6)

At the 'cutting edge' perhaps, but ICTs are very much only part of both the 'problem' and 'solution' posed by Centrelink. At a theoretical level, the public service model represented by Centrelink represents something of an apotheosis for the capabilities enabled by, and embodied in, concepts of IM. It is a model of service delivery that is, as far as is legally and practically possible, boundary-free, in which cross-agency applications become genuinely possible; the traditional model of public service delivery, where 'one size fits all', has been replaced by something that is much more client-centric, with information resource access and sharing at the centre of all processes which serve to make this possible. However, it is perhaps wise to caution that the example of Centrelink should be viewed very much as a 'work in progress', the best opportunity that we have in a global context to examine the ways in which IM strategy has been deployed in a test-bed scenario, where our 'laboratory' is a major global economy.

So what specific points can we take from the Centrelink example which will help to establish a road map of good IM practice for other public sector contexts? Well, in the first instance there is the largely generalisable issue that arises from public sector and indeed 'political' time-scales often being somewhat constrained in nature. Thus, the major refocusing of service delivery pattern that was represented by Centrelink was driven forward in a time period of less than one year, from first draft policy document to actual launch, with ambitious goals articulated, often with some degree of vagueness, in 1997 and expected to be delivered on in 1998. So if we consider the draft policy statement of August 1997, we can see that 'key result areas' in respect of service delivery were anticipated in a number of information-intensive areas:

Simplify Processes

• building integrated employment services – registration, assessment and referral systems;
• examine simplification and integration of decision-making processes;
• review resource allocation process to ensure flexibility and appropriate delegation;
• search for new technologies to assist with service delivery.

Quality Service

• establish and implement a national quality framework;
• develop benchmark procedures;
• provide a single point of contact for customers;
• ensure accurate, equitable, unbiased, consistent decision making;
• encourage customers to provide direct feedback on service delivery decisions;

- implement arrangements for advising customers of decisions on their entitlements;
- develop and implement national service delivery business plans which support Agency goals.

Marketing

- active marketing of achievement and potential of the Agency;
- identify and pursue avenues for marketing agency skills, knowledge and technology both nationally and internationally;
- all managers to actively participate in community liaison.
                                    (Department for Social Security 1997: 12)

The time-frame suggested, and indeed permitted, to Centrelink staff to bring about the major changes and to meet the challenges alluded to in this draft policy statement would, even if resources were unlimited, represent a considerable undertaking. Add to this the fact that the changes envisaged were profound both for those who had been employed within a variety of distinct operating units and also for the end-user, who had been accustomed to a multiple-gateway method of interacting with government services, and one can begin to understand why Centrelink is best described as 'a work in progress'.

From an IM perspective one should ask: among all of the many 'theme teams' that were put in place to deliver the 'key result areas' outlined above, was there an IM monitoring team which operated across 'themes' to ensure that issues of good practice and common operating standards were adhered to? The answer, not surprising given our previous reflections upon predilections for subsuming issues of IM within an overtly technological framework, is that issues around information sharing, information security and end-user access were generally discussed under the 'umbrella' theme of information and communications technology. Given that we have already argued that there is much that can be lost through the adoption of such an approach, perhaps the first and most valuable lesson from which we can then build our model of good practice is to acknowledge that IM is likely to have resonance and impact within multiple layers of a public sector change agenda, of which the ICT component is only one part. To be effective, therefore, IM identification and audit procedures need to be introduced from the outset, with both a capability and an expectation that they will 'join-up' in a coherent framework that positions the critical public sector information resource at the centre of the change management process.

Information audit

The concept of auditing is well established in respect of organisational financial operations, where there is both a legal and an economic imperative to examine the way in which specified resources and assets are managed. However, there has been a discernible movement, particularly evident in respect of the growth in interest of quality management and business process reengineering techniques, to broaden the scope of the term 'audit' to allow it to encompass an examination and itemisation of other, non-financial, resources and activities found within all organisations. Perhaps the best known of such audit applications are those which relate to the training function and which form part of an explicit requirement in the United Kingdom for the award of Investor in People, and those around environmental standards and practices as articulated by the International Standards Organisation.

However, an audit of the training function, or of procurement activities or environmental factors, represents an interaction with something that is in some way 'visible'. When we move to suggest that a critical aspect of audit processes should be a regular review of information assets, there are immediate problems around identifying what it is that you are auditing, how you actually measure or define the 'worth' of that information and what, having grappled with these problems, you are actually going to do with the outcomes of your audit. By focusing upon these questions, the intention here is to demonstrate that the adoption and maintenance of information auditing approaches and methodologies represent critical first steps in moving beyond the rhetoric of IM policies, ensuring that strategies are capable of being actioned and giving cause for optimism that Strassman's somewhat pessimistic view may be amended: 'Insofar as the contributions of people, information and knowledge are concerned, the financial statistics remain silent because none of these contributions to creating greater economic value are recognised in generally accepted accounting principles' (Manasco 1996: 1).

Probably the most important conceptual element of information auditing is the need to clearly set out the purpose and value of undertaking such a potentially time-consuming and costly activity. The reason for stating that this is primarily an issue of 'concept' rather than communication – initially at least – is that it is highly probable that the audit champion or leader will be promoting what is often an unfamiliar way of requiring the organisation to assess or measure 'value'. Perhaps ironically, it is a mode of thought which is likely to be more readily accommodated and welcomed by public sector managers than it has yet proven to be in the commercial sector, where an explicit 'bottom line' provides the anchor and guidance system for almost all business activities.

Fundamentally, what information auditing exists to do is to demonstrate opportunities and rationale for reducing 'waste', perhaps defined as duplication of activity or the continuance of outmoded and unnecessary work practices, by pointing to the information flows and processes which sustain and support such activities and which might otherwise remain invisible to the wider organisation. So in this respect, information audits can be said to have the potential to leverage the efficiency of an operation, possibly resulting in reduced costs and perhaps also an enhanced level of service to the end-user, be they an internal public service customer or the citizen as external customer. A further function of audit activity is to stimulate the asking of questions: in respect of information they can usually be categorised very simply as 'why?' and 'why not?' So, for instance, why do two sections within one government department collect, organise and archive identical information items? And why don't they share this information across their notional boundaries? Are other departments gathering the same information, and is it actually required? And, ultimately, what value does it add to the operation of the department or agency and to their end-users?

The concept of the information audit is, of course, further complicated by the fact that what you are often dealing with is essentially intangible: you may not necessarily be able to see it, touch it or count it, but in order to harness it you know one thing – you have to understand it. Kaplan and Norton, in their influential and ground-breaking work on the development of a 'balanced score-card' for assessing and moving forward organisational performance, provide a useful summary of the challenges facing those charged with moving forward the management of intangible assets:

> Today's managers recognize the impact that measures have on performance. But they rarely think of measurement as an essential part of their strategy. For example, executives may introduce new strategies and innovative operating processes, intended to achieve breakthrough performance, then continue to use the same short-term financial indicators that have been used for decades, measures like return on investment … These managers not only fail to introduce new measures to monitor new goals and processes but also to question whether or not their old measures are relevant to their new initiatives.
>
> (Kaplan and Norton 1993: 134)

Public sector organisations are typically structured to manage the tangible assets they hold, for example their buildings, computer hardware and structures and hierarchies relating to their people. However, such assets represent only a tiny proportion of the 'worth' and activity of something such as social security and benefits activity, or education, or transport and treasury operations. The process of public administration is fundamentally a service industry and, as such, its proportion of intangible assets heavily outweighs the tangible; yet only now, at the outset of the twenty-first century, are we beginning to see any real acknowledgement that this is the case.

Unfortunately, as yet there is no credible or robust model of information auditing which can be adopted in an 'off the shelf' manner and deployed without considerable need for customisation and high degrees of expertise. However, there are some generic principles around audit focus and design which may usefully be adapted or indeed adopted across a range of public sector scenarios. These involve three key stages: identification of audit purpose; choice of audit methodology; and reporting of outcomes.

Identification of audit purpose

It is never going to be enough to say 'we need to audit our information assets', because, after all, to a large part of the audit constituency this is likely to be a meaningless statement. In order to design the audit methodology and to gain support for its resourcing, there is a need to be clear in all communications regarding what it is that is being looked at, and with what purpose in mind. Brooking and Motta put forward a useful but largely commercial-sector oriented taxonomy of intellectual capital, which with some significant amendments provides a useful template for ensuring that, from the outset, the information audit process is focused upon the needs of the organisation and of key groups within it (Brooking and Motta 1996: 4). It should also be recognised that, for such a template to be used realistically, it should be capable of demonstrating value and relevance when deployed at both the macro level, which might be across one or several functions of public administration as in the case of Centrelink, or in a micro-operating environment, which might involve perhaps only one small sub-function or geographic location of the public service in question.

How are the information processes supporting the achievement of service goals?

Through understanding strategies and ongoing change agenda that impact upon the organisational culture and priorities, information processing activities and their content should be reviewed in respect of the contribution that they are, or might be, capable of making to the achievement of change. Where resources are finite, and they almost always will be, this is the opportunity to look at the way in which information processes operate and relate to each other, and to consider the potential for achieving cost efficiencies through reductions in duplication. There should also be consideration of legacies from past structures and informed judgements about whether the information processes that they have bequeathed are actually necessary. In the case of Centrelink, it might well have been a useful exercise to have mapped existing information processes against the needs of the new organisation and its goals: the benefit is that such a task highlights gaps and mismatches and can help to lay the foundations for a model of operation that is related to actual service needs.

The term 'mapping', when used here, refers to a commonly used work-flow analysis technique which can be successfully utilised within an information audit scenario. What it serves to do is to show, through graphic representation of flows, where duplication of information activity is taking place, where information is flowing to, what is in essence a 'dead end', and where instances of information overload may be occurring. Specific software packages to support this activity are beginning to reach the market and represent a potentially useful tool in the hands of trained personnel. However, where information 'maps' are used to demonstrate a business case for change it is possible that they can serve to confuse and distract from the key activities being promoted. The primary reason for this, as can be seen in Figure 3.1, is that an information mapping exercise can result in a complex and dense representation of a given scenario, which is useful in its 'raw' state for supporting analysis activity but potentially dangerous if used as a main mode of communication of key audit findings to key interest groups. If a mapping representation is deemed to be useful in conveying outcomes or providing indicators for change, it may well be that a simplified map, focused upon illustrating key themes, will best serve the cause of IM, as opposed to one depicting every single information flow in detail.

What information is required for successful organisational reengineering?

One of the few certainties facing any public sector organisation is that change and change pressures are an ever-present part of life. The imperative here is that, in auditing your information assets on a regular basis, change should proceed on the basis of a sound understanding of many critical factors which might otherwise be (and in reality often are) overlooked. When embarking upon change strategies for information-intensive processes such as benefits payments, there is a need to have a fundamental understanding of the information elements that make up the claim, including processing and payment aspects, and identifying and analysing as many possible variables around this interaction as resources permit. By investing time in this activity, the likelihood of achieving a change that actually works, where problems and allied wastage of time and further resources are minimised, is considerably enhanced.

A recommendation that may result from focus upon this particular question is the need for some index of information holdings and processes to be held and maintained on an organisation-wide basis. With the developments in Intranet technologies it is likely that such an index would be stored electronically and accessible throughout the organisation, although possibly with differing levels of security access. Audit activity, taking place as part of an ongoing programme, would serve to ensure that information items indexed were appropriately classified and to monitor issues of inclusion and deletion on a regular basis. An index of information assets, be they internally or externally generated, is likely to provide one of the most useful tools currently available in moving forward issues of IM in public service organisations.

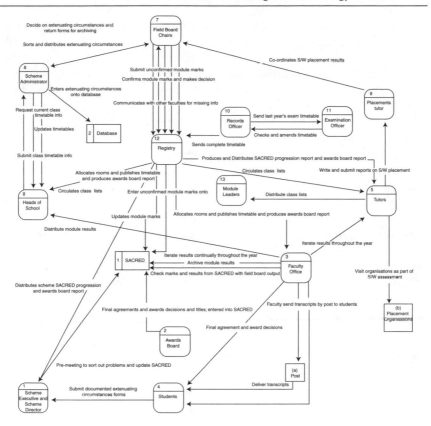

Figure 3.1   Example of an information audit map

In the context of driving forward change, you need also to be looking at the information 'roles and responsibilities' that are evident in the existing organisation. Who is responsible for managing the gathering and use of key information items? Are there any quality measures or checks in place? Where does responsibility for archiving and deletion lie? If the key audit question here is to ask what information is needed for change to be successful, then the subsidiary issue must surely be to ascertain who is responsible for it. And if through audit of existing structures you are able to identify blockages or impediments to necessary information flowing, as our now familiar adage would have it, to the right place, at the right time and in the right format, then the task becomes a structural one: removing 'blockages' and ensuring that information flows are appropriate to present and emerging organisational needs. However, such an approach makes one important although potentially problematic assumption, and that is that there will be a widespread recognition of exactly what information is required to support and drive forward change.

When you are carrying out an audit, what you are focusing on is almost always what actually *exists*; to assume, in the case of information, that this represents what you actually *need* can be rather dangerous. Probably the best advice that one can offer in this context is to concentrate planning activities on building change scenarios – sometimes referred to as the 'heaven and hell' school of management! By doing this you involve key people in making informed predictions, or – as they are sometimes described, with rather more optimism than scientific rationale – 'models' of the future, based upon what is perceived to be the ideal outcome of change and how this might look in practice. Conversely, it is also useful to give some consideration to the very worst outcome that might be predicted. You can begin to build a map of what information you actually need to make the 'heaven' scenario a reality and to avoid the pitfalls of the 'hell' that you have modelled. Such a scenario and its information requirements can then be mapped against what you have currently, which you already know about because you have audited existing practice, and from this you can look at the way in which reengineering of information processes needs to be actioned. Too frequently, this critical element of the change process is neglected or given only partial consideration, and the result is all too often costly and wasteful delay and service shortfall.

Do we know the value of our information?

Questions around information value are extremely problematic in all sectors of the economy, largely because it is so difficult to assign any balance sheet figure to what such assets are actually worth. In research carried out at the University of North London which involved a review of a sample of annual reports for 1994/5 of the FTSE 500 companies, it was found that even in what might be deemed 'information intensive' service industries, no valuation was assigned to the importance of information holdings, and indeed scarcely any mention was made of it at all (Milner 1997a). This was a finding supported by a more broadly focused study undertaken by The Technology Broker company, which found that, in a sample of 226 of the FTSE-quoted companies, only 76 per cent made any mention in annual reports of intangible assets; where reference was made, it was to brand value and the importance of goodwill (Brooking and Motta 1996: 1). In a public service context there has been a still more marked absence of focus upon the potential worth of information assets, particularly in the ability of their effective and sometimes innovative use to deliver better and more cost-efficient services. It is probably true to say that among major global economies it is only the government of Canada which has devoted significant research effort towards addressing this issue; a 1993 research report states: 'In a time of increasing competition for decreasing funds, any previously held assumptions about the value of information can no longer be left unchallenged' (Menou 1993: iv).

So what, then, do we need to challenge in respect of information valuation? We know that it is difficult, we know also that it is a neglected area of management, but what does it actually involve? Probably the most influential academic operating within this area of valuation is Glazer, who since the early 1990s has been working on the development of what he describes as the 'information value chain' (Glazer 1993: 100). Using the continuum discussed in Chapter 1, which sees data taking on the characteristics of information through the processes of collection and structuring, and through analysis, interpretation and use resulting in knowledge, Glazer puts forward the goal 'to capture the value of the information at each point along the chain' (Glazer 1993: 100). In order to do this effectively, he further cautions that we must fundamentally understand the 'uniqueness' of information assets:

> Any discussion of an information or knowledge theory of value must begin with an analysis of the peculiar attributes of information as a commodity. The typical economic good displays such properties as divisibility, appropriability, scarcity and decreasing returns on use. By contrast, information as a commodity differs from the typical good in that (1) it is not easily divisible or appropriable (i.e., either I have it or you have it); (2) it is not inherently scarce (although it is often perishable); and (3) it may not exhibit decreasing returns to use, but often in fact increases in value the more it is used; (4) unlike other commodities, which are non-renewable and with exceptions depletable, information is self-regenerative or feeds on itself so that the identification of a new piece of knowledge immediately creates both the demand and conditions for production of subsequent pieces.
>
> (Glazer 1993: 101)

Therefore the challenge presented in moving to adopt an audit approach is to ensure that all those involved understand the complexity and potential benefits of the undertaking. Perhaps the opening position is to acknowledge first that the majority of public services are, as we have stated, information-intensive operations; this in itself may be a major point of clarification for many senior managers and politicians. From this position of recognition, perhaps the most easily accessible way in which to discuss issues of value is to focus on the negative that can result from having only a partial understanding of the information items held – primarily matters such as opportunities for inefficiency, service failure and perhaps even fraud, and the security issues that may surround them. One relatively simple indicator of information value is to attempt to evaluate the replacement value of certain categories of information. Another might be to calculate potential efficiency savings that might result from information sharing.

Focusing upon matters of information value with an evidence-base provided by audit data represents the best and perhaps the only way of achieving senior-level commitment to principles of IM. The methodology for demonstrating this value is far more complex than any mathematical model or equation that might be deployed when dealing with more tangible assets; however, the cost benefit implications, never yet fully explored by a national or regional government, are likely to be very considerable. This is why matters of valuation should be raised at the outset of any audit planning activity.

Audit methodology

After considering the major questions that should be asked in respect of effective identification of audit purpose, there is then a need to consider what methodologies might be available and how they could best be deployed within a public service context. Having achieved appropriate management commitment for an audit to be conducted, the questions of what is to be done and who is to do it present themselves. The first consideration is to clearly define the area of service to be audited and to delineate whether the scope of the audit is to be inclusive or to focus on one or more specific types of information item. A pilot study remains the best way of trailing methodologies to be deployed in a resource- and time-limited manner, permitting further review, training and revision of processes to take place prior to any larger-scale audit.

In an ideal operating scenario, a team of dedicated information auditors would be deployed across functions or departments. The value of such an approach is, of course, that expertise is built and targeted, as has been demonstrated in the UK National Health Service with its teams of clinical auditors working on a regional basis. However, as the concept of information auditing is so very new and the pool of experienced personnel so very limited, it is likely that the first public service organisations to recognise the value of such a process are likely to be found to rely on one of two approaches: it may be that external consultants are contracted to undertake such work or, perhaps more likely, it could be that the champion of this approach will have, in the first instance at least, to draw together a team of people to work on a 'project' basis. In the commercial sector it has been interesting to note that champions of information auditing have been drawn from a diverse range of functional specialisms, with marketing and finance appearing to show particularly strong interest in the concept.

Having identified the area to be audited and the team of people to be involved the basis upon which the methodology is designed can usefully emerge from the asking of five key questions, which Earl presents as his model of 'information equity':

- Have we got the information we need?
- Do we know what information we have got?

- Do we use the information we have?
- Is the information we have as effective as we want?
- Is our information processing economically viable?

(Earl 1995: 6)

Such a question-based approach is extremely useful inasmuch as it serves to focus the mind of the auditor or team on key specific issues to which answers can be sought through the effective gathering of relevant data. It also suggests what is likely to emerge in practice anyway: that for information auditing to be undertaken successfully, the information items need to be broken down into manageable categories, with aggregation across items and functions taking place when appropriate.

The gathering of sufficient data to provide a platform of response to these questions is unlikely to emerge from the deployment of only one methodology, and it is also highly unlikely that a high proportion of this data can be generated electronically without the need for considerable human intervention. As was suggested previously when considering the first of Earl's questions (have we got the information we need?) there is an imperative to engage key stakeholders in some discussion, whether it be structured, by means of a questionnaire-based methodology, or the rather more free-flowing scenario-building approach discussed previously in this chapter. Whatever approach is used, the role of the audit team is to ask and to challenge; a deceptively simple question around information need can result in a whole spectrum of subjective responses being returned, many of which may be based rather more upon personal preference than on actual requirement.

Itemising categories of information can be a profoundly illuminating experience, particularly when such data are measured against what is established as realistic *need*. Audit of existing information holdings is, initially at least, often a time-consuming exercise; an audit team is building a picture of what exists, and this may be complex, available to few or many, and called different things by different constituencies within the workplace.

A further metric that presents itself for consideration at this stage is the allied factor of *usage*. Having established that an information item exists, for audit purposes it is then necessary to assign it some classification of use: for example, in a benefits payment scenario it might be that client claim details are to be classified as having high intensity of usage and widespread inter-office access, whereas information on staff sickness has medium intensity of usage, with only limited access by a small number of managers. These three considerations form what is referred to as an information audit loop, which focuses upon *need*, *existing holdings* and *use* and provides a basis for further investigation and particularisation of the audit function in alignment with the underpinning goals of the process, be they simply ensuring that existing processes are better understood or – perhaps more likely – enabling a meaningful contribution to be made to improvements in overall organisational performance.

Earl suggests two further dimensions which should be considered along-side the basic audit loop: the measurement of information 'effectiveness', and the 'processing' costs. For these two considerations to be successfully assimilated into the audit function, there is an absolute requirement that the data on need, identification and use is already in place, for it is informed knowledge of these considerations which will enable indicators of effective-ness and cost to be framed within an accurate representation of specific IM situations. The question of effectiveness is paradoxically both a straightfor-ward and complex undertaking. In respect of adopting a sound methodological framework for its measurement, it is likely that the most useful way forward is a matrix or index of effectiveness factors, representing graded categories or indicators against which information performance can be classified.

The IMPACT Programme 'health index' is useful when considering moving forward the audit work represented by the baseline audit loop model. It is primarily a tool which focuses upon providing an indication of performance and, rather like better-known models such as the European Quality Model, it was intended that the index should provide a basis for both internal and external benchmarking activities in relation to IM. To understand the way in which the index is structured and scores assigned, we need to understand that, in the case of this particular tool, indicators have been constructed in alignment with the Hawley Committee recommenda-tions, discussed in Chapters 1 and 2 (IMPACT Ltd 1994). Thus they are perhaps open to the criticism of being somewhat narrow in scope, if the intention of the audit process is to encompass all levels of IM within an organisation. However, as a template of what good practice might look like in achieving a meaningful representation of information effectiveness, this inherently flexible approach represents ground-breaking work in this area and is capable of the wider adaptation required to ensure a tool of value to public sector organisations. If we consider the structure of the index in rela-tion to just one 'indicator', that which requires that 'all information is marked with identification, source, date of last use, and confidentiality clas-sification', we will see in Table 3.1 that five measures of practice and effectiveness are set out:

Table 3.1 Impact information management health index

The Board should satisfy itself that its own business is conducted so that:

1 The information it uses is necessary and sufficient for its purpose.

1.1 Positive, formal review within last 12 months of Board's corporate calendar and information

100%	75%	50%	25%	0%
There has been a positive review of the corporate calendar and Board information within the last twelve months, necessary changes to Board papers have been agreed, and actions have been taken accordingly	There has been a positive review of the corporate calendar and Board information, but not within the last twelve months and/or necessary changes to Board papers have not yet been agreed, and/or not yet implemented	The importance of the corporate calendar and the information required to support has been recognised as important by the Board but no comprehensive plan exists to review the situation	Some discussion has taken place and some changes have been made to Board information on an ad hoc basis in the last twelve months but no review in the context of Information as an Asset has been agreed	The issue of adequate Board information is not recognised as important, evidenced by the lack of discussion on Board information within the last two years

2 It is aware of and properly advised on the information aspects of all the subjects on its agenda.

2.1 Nominated Executive Director responsible for information aspects, external advice received if required

100%	75%	50%	25%	0%
A director has been nominated as the authority on information management and terms of reference agreed, external advice has been discussed and actioned as necessary within the last year, and discussion of information asset affairs is routine	A director has been nominated as the authority on information management and terms of reference agreed, but external advice has not been discussed, and/or discussion of information asset affairs is not yet routine	It has been recognised that a director should be nominated as the authority on information management but no plan is in place to achieve this	Without specific consideration of information as an asset, directors nevertheless have responsibilities which cover some, but not all, of the requirements	The issue of Board responsibility for information assets is not regarded as important, evidenced by no discussion having taken place nor action taken to identify responsibility

2.2 Insistence that information aspects are specifically included in all relevant Board papers

100%	75%	50%	25%	0%
All plans, budgets, investment and divestiture proposals, and other documents considered by the Board, adequately cover information aspects as a normal routine, there is a quality check in place, and the results are satisfactory	Instructions have been given on how all Board papers will cover information aspects but these have not yet been fully implemented, and/or there is no quality check, and/or the results of checks are not satisfactory	It has been agreed that information aspects should always be covered in relevant Board papers but no adequate plan to achieve this is yet in place	While information aspects are not required to be covered in Board papers, the importance of information assets has been recognised and discussed in at least one issue before the Board in the last year	The Board does not recognise the importance of information aspects in its affairs, evidenced by lack of discussion in any of its affairs

3 Its own use of information, collectively and individually, complies with applicable laws, regulations and recognised ethical standards.

3.1 *Documented list, reviewed within the last twelve months, circulated to all directors of information-related regulations together with a simple explanation of non-compliance*

100%	75%	50%	25%	0%
An adequate, up-to-date list of regulations covering directors' responsibilities related to information assets exists, has been circulated to directors within the last year, has a simple explanation of the consequences of non-compliance, and directors have expressed their satisfaction	An adequate, up-to-date list of regulations covering directors' responsibilities related to information assets exists, but has not been circulated to directors within the last year, and/or has not got a simple explanation of the consequences of non-compliance, and/or directors have not yet expressed satisfaction	The importance of having a list of regulations affecting directors' responsibilities related to information assets is recognised but no plan to achieve this is yet in place	A list of regulations affecting directors' responsibilities exists which covers some, but not all, matters related to information assets	The issue of compliance to laws and regulations is not regarded as important, evidenced by there being no list of regulations related to directors' responsibilities

The Board should determine the organisations policy for information assets and identify how compliance with that policy will be measured and reviewed, including:

3.2 Existence of an information policy, giving clear guidance on all information aspects and stating clearly which are reserved to the Board

100%	75%	50%	25%	0%
An information policy exists, covering all aspects of the Hawley Agenda, which states what is reserved for decision by the Board, has been widely circulated in the last year, is included in company training, and checks within the last year have shown a high level of awareness	An information policy exists, covering all aspects of the Hawley Agenda, which states what is reserved for decision by the Board, but it has not been circulated within the last year, and/or is not included in company training, and/or there is no evidence of widespread awareness	The importance of having an information policy, covering all aspects of the Hawley Agenda, is recognised, but no plan to achieve this is yet in place	No comprehensive information policy exists, but some aspects required in an information policy are contained in other policy documents, except in the IS facility which, measured on its own, would score at least 75 per cent	The issue of an information policy is not recognised as important, evidenced by no information policy existing anywhere in the organisation

3.3 Process in place and properly resourced for measuring compliance with the information policy and regular reports received during the last twelve months

100%	75%	50%	25%	0%
A process is in place and resourced (e.g. the internal audit department) to provide effective reporting on compliance with the Board's policy on information	A process has been defined, but not fully resourced for reporting on compliance with the Board's policy on information, and/or regular reports have not been received in the last year, and/or the results have not been satisfactory	It has been recognised that measurement of compliance with information policy is important but no adequate plan to achieve this is yet in place	Reports to the Board on compliance with some aspects of information management policy is covered within other compliance measurement, but there is no cohesive report on information management	The issue of compliance with information policy is not regarded as important, evidenced by no adequate compliance measurement with information management policy anywhere in the organisation

4 The identification of information assets and the classification into those of value and importance that merit special attention and those that do not.

4.1 An up-to-date information asset register exists showing the relative importance of information assets and their confidentiality classification

100%	75%	50%	25%	0%
A practical and effective information asset register exists, has been reviewed within the last year, and has been approved by the Board, which shows assets which are to be regarded as valuable and at least indicates their relative importance and their confidentiality classifications	A practical and effective information asset register exists, but has not been reviewed within the last year, and/or has not been approved by the Board, and/or does not at least indicate relative importance and/or confidentiality classifications	The importance of compiling an information asset register is recognised but no comprehensive plan to achieve this is yet in place	Some information assets are recognised and managed either separately or in other documents, but coverage is not complete, and there is no information asset register except in the IS facility which, if measured on its own, would score at least 75 per cent	The concept of managing information as an asset is not recognised as important, evidenced by no information asset register existing or contemplated

4.2 All information is marked with identification, source, date of last issue, and confidentiality classification

100%	75%	50%	25%	0%
All information, and each separable subset of information, is identified by a source, date of last issue and implied or explicit confidentiality classification and checks within the last year have shown a high level of compliance	Instructions exist for all information to be identified by a source, date of last issue and confidentiality classification, but this is not fully implemented, and/or there are inadequate checks and/or checks show non-compliance	The appropriate marking of all information assets is recognised as important but no adequate plan to achieve this is yet in place	Some, but not all, information is identified by a source, date of last issue and confidentiality classification, as part of other schemes, except in the IS department which, if measured on its own, would score at least 75 per cent	The appropriate marking of information has not been recognised as an important issue, evidenced by no systematic scheme

4.3 *Information assets are required to have specific mention in strategy, planning, budgeting and reporting documents throughout the organisation*

100%	75%	50%	25%	0%
All aspects of the management of information assets are specifically covered, with equal emphasis to tangible assets, in plans, budgets and performance reports to management and to the Board and checks show compliance throughout the organisation	All aspects of the management of information assets are required to be covered, with equal emphasis to tangible assets, in plans, budgets and performance reports, but coverage is incomplete and/or checking is inadequate or checks reveal that compliance is not complete	It is recognised that all aspects of the management of information assets should be included in strategic plans, budgets and performance reports, but no adequate plan to achieve this is yet in place	Some, but not all, aspects of the management of information assets are contained in some strategic plans and budgets on an ad hoc basis, there is no overall requirement to cover management assets, except in the IS facility which, if measured on its own, would score at least 75 per cent	The management of information assets is not recognised as an important issue, evidenced by there being no emphasis on planning and reporting

Source: ©1996 IMPACT Ltd

Assessment of performance against the indicators is made against five scoring point ranges. The individual or team charged with conducting this measure makes an assessment based upon identification of the lowest scoring point which can be held to be true for the organisation or function being assessed. Thus, where a score between 0 per cent and 25 per cent is assigned, it may be assumed that both IM practice and effectiveness can be deemed to be 'poor'; between 25 per cent and 50 per cent the assessment indicates 'fair' performance; 50 per cent up to 75 per cent is 'good'; and obviously the pinnacle of IM achievement is 'excellent', indicated by a score of 75 per cent to 100 per cent. What is particularly useful in respect of this health index approach is the fact that it recommends that indicators, or 'symptoms' as they are more correctly described, are provided in relation to each of the scoring bands. Framed as no more than short descriptive paragraphs, they provide an accessible mode of engaging a wider constituency in making an assessment of the practice of IM within an organisation. Thus, if, after the initial pilot stage recommended at the outset of the consideration of information audit practice, it is decided to move the process out into the organisation more generally, then the development of indicators and associated symptoms by specialist teams may lead to the creation of a user-friendly and effective mode of self-assessment.

The final issue associated with the audit process is that of considering the costs and benefits of existing practice, sometimes referred to in the literature as the search for information 'value'. This represents potentially the most complex information audit procedure, and it is one which it is difficult to incorporate within any index mechanism. The audit loop which was introduced previously, and particularly any mapping exercises associated with its deployment, represents the best opportunity for gauging the scale and scope of the range of processes associated with IM within any organisation. This in itself may be a revelatory exercise, for while Earl suggests that the question we must focus upon is 'Is our information processing economically viable?' (Earl 1995: 1), in the public sector this question may be better phrased as 'Are all of our information processes necessary, and do we know what they actually cost us?' Such a perspective, while far from an exact science, can provide pointers as to where costs are accruing, be they measured in the use of time, unnecessary pressure on ICT functions, duplication of effort, or even lost opportunities, to name only four examples. What we are working towards, as Earl suggests, is the achievement of an IM perspective where:

Increasingly there will be organization-wide measures to measure collective competence in the ability to use information. Such measures may help raise consciousness of how important it is to be able to use the critical asset of the information age. For one of the most practical measures of information value is information use. And one of the biggest constraints on information use is information capacity. Use is not just a proxy measure for information value. Use releases value.

(Earl 1995: 12)

Information audit: a checklist for success

We have established that information audit can be a critical tool in moving from a policy position on IM to one of implementation and action. However, there are inherent dangers associated with any 'faddish' adoption of this technique, which would see it deployed once and then be replaced by the next 'fad' recommended by management gurus. For it to be successful, it has to become embedded in the life cycle of organisational work practice, managed through clearly articulated lines of responsibility and supported through appropriate education and training programmes. As with other types of audit, it is a representation of what you have and what you do with it over a given time period. As such, it forms the basis of an informed under-standing of information strengths and weaknesses, the former suggesting themselves for further exploitation, the latter requiring remedial action which may see change or deletion of the process or items.

On the basis of this recognition of the potential role and value of commit-ting to an information audit, it is possible to put forward a checklist of audit activities which, taken as a whole, should make a significant contribution to the achievement of organisational 'value added'. The first area of focus must be *defining the purpose of the information audit*: by this we mean clearly articu-lating the three stages of the audit loop in language which reflects the existing operational make-up of the audit subject. One of the most common difficulties associated with this stage is the lack of common operating language, both within and across public service organisations. Therefore, one of the critical first steps for an individual or team charged with the design and operationalisa-tion of such an activity is to ensure that those who ask and answer key questions actually understand one another. As yet there is little evidence of common operating languages being prioritised by public service organisations on a stand-alone basis, and still less of any cross-organisational work based on agreed common operating terminology.

This issue has been raised by the International Council for Information Technology in Government Administration (ICA), which stated that 'managing the new, cross agency systems for improved data sharing and data management was one of the top issues facing ICA member countries' (ICA 1998a: 5). Although couched in terms which may be more obviously syner-gous with issues of IS than with IM, the principle discussed is undoubtedly pertinent to our concern to minimise the difficulties caused to IM, and to support audit processes in particular, by the lack of common 'information' languages found within the public service globally.

Work on defining and then communicating the purpose of the information audit can in itself provide a useful data-gathering opportunity. In an ideal scenario, for audit practitioners to deliver greatest value to this process, public service organisations would be well advised to put in place dedicated audit teams, whose purpose over time is to provide the architecture and materials for the achievement of an IM-focused organisation. While we have said earlier in this chapter that the reality, when audit approaches are adopted, is for senior managers to take a cautious project-based approach probably characterised by a number of small pilot studies, the reality in the longer term is that this activity should not be viewed as an ad hoc one-off experiment. Critical to the ongoing success of information audit will be the way in which it manages to become embedded in the annual life cycle of public service operations.

Thus, for information audit to deliver hoped-for returns, it has to be understood at a senior level and resourced appropriately and on an ongoing basis. The role of the IM champion is critical in moving this forward and in ensuring that the rationale and positive outcomes of moving to such an approach are raised through all appropriate channels. One potential avenue for moving to a position of widespread support for aspects of IM, particularly audit activity, is to research practice in other service-based organisations, particularly those in the commercial sector. The rationale for this is, of course, to highlight the benefits accruing to other types of organisation from the adoption of specific IM tools, but also, perhaps more cynically, to tap into a wider and still prevalent perception, particularly on the part of many politicians, that public sector practice still has much to learn from its commercial sector counterparts. Particularly interesting in this respect might be some focus upon the emerging role and status of a chief information officer (CIO) role within many commercial sector organisations, so that at board level there is an individual charged with ensuring that all IM functions operate to their very best potential.

Moving audit activity out across an organisation as vast in scale as the United States Internal Revenue Service or the UK National Health Service, or indeed the Australian example of Centrelink, is clearly a massive undertaking. This kind of undertaking should only be resourced and actioned on the basis of clearly expressed objectives, time-scales and performance indicators – omitting these in any organisational process is to invite dissipation of effort and waste of resources. Thus, evaluation of audit process and outcomes should be viewed as a further critical factor in ensuring that such activities retain relevance and value to the organisation.

Fundamentally, however, what all of these factors and processes relating to audit and 'valuation' methodologies should facilitate is the achievement of cross-departmental or agency information sharing. The ICA report cited previously suggests that it is only by moving to such a position that fundamental and positive change in public services can actually be achieved, and that in order to do this a number of key issues must be considered:

Integrated service delivery in the 'milieu' of an all-pervasive infrastructure extending to the homes and public places, the service extensions to traditional transaction systems offered by the Internet and Intranets and the harnessing of common elements of data and information relationships across agencies. A 'single window' for citizen and business interface with government. Behind that single window, processes must also be rationalized, along with benefits and revenue programmes and the dissemination of information.

(ICA 1998a: 5)

It is only through knowing what information public service organisations have, what they currently do with it and what they actually need that these issues can begin to be realistically addressed. A move to information auditing, with an allied focus upon a meaningful definition of the value of information assets to a public sector organisation or function, provides the building blocks for the achievement of 'information age government'. However, for such an approach to be successful certain factors must be regarded as critical, and these can be summarised as the DREAD components of information audit and valuation return on investment:

Define the purpose and remit of the audit in appropriate terminology;
Resource your audit processes adequately and carry out pilot studies;
Evaluate the efficacy of both audit process and outcome arising from pilot phases and amend as required;
Advocate within and across organisations the benefits accruing from this approach;
Deploy as widely as possible to ensure maximum returns.

These factors, when taken together, can be said to represent the building blocks of the achievement of an IM business case for public service organisations. The key to success lies in successfully designing and carrying out appropriate information audits which link firmly to ongoing organisational change agenda. Indeed, in a wider context they must also link to the rationale underpinning global re-evaluation of public service structures and modes of operation, such as the ambitious and innovative Centrelink example discussed in this chapter.

Chapter 4

Knowledge management

So far we have considered mainly issues and methodologies around the specific subject of information management. However, from the outset it was made clear that although the journey towards the adoption of successful IM practices can itself offer considerable opportunities to achieve improvement, there was a further stage on this journey which has the potential to bring still greater rewards: the destination in this case is the achievement of 'knowledge management' (KM). First gaining widespread recognition as a management term in the late 1990s, KM invites, and receives, a wide range of responses from both academics and practitioners. The spectrum of view ranges from the overwhelmingly positive:

> Knowledge Management is big business. It has been flaunted as the differentiator between companies, the means to gaining competitive advantage. As the information society continues to grow exponentially, so have the opportunities to gather and use knowledge to optimum effect.
>
> (Rock 1998: 4)

through to the more cynical and negative, expressed here in terms of 'intellectual capital' (IC), a term which is often used interchangeably with KM in the literature: 'at best IC will bore you to death. At worst, IC is a potential Trojan Horse for those who want stakeholders, not shareholders, to control our companies, and social agendas, not performance to drive business decisions' (Rutledge 1997: 10).

So, having considered these almost polarised views of the value of KM and its components, what is it? The creation and use of knowledge can be said to underpin the development of mankind, for it is linked, critically, to the ability of humans to learn, to interpret and to make judgements. As such, we should acknowledge that there is nothing particularly revolutionary about the principles of KM. It is about ensuring that your human resources are being utilised to greatest effect, the intention being to maximise the value of this asset group, just as we have previously discussed ways in which information assets, when properly understood and focused, can be harnessed to add value to the organisation and its operations.

To seek a precise definition of what is meant by KM is to invite confusion, for unhelpfully, just as for IM, there remains a stubborn body of thought which relates KM entirely to ICT applications and primarily to database exploitation. An example of this view is put forward by Anthes, who defines KM as: 'policies, procedures and technologies employed for operating a continuously updated linked pair of networked databases' (Anthes 1991:28). Such a view, while undoubtedly pointing towards one application of KM tools, is far from a complete or indeed helpful definition of what we are considering here. For KM, as we shall move to define it, can be said to offer modern public services one of the most exciting and far-reaching opportunities for the achievement of organisational and cultural change that we have yet witnessed. However, there is a real danger that the hype and hyperbole surrounding it will only serve to diminish its influence and create a climate of cynicism in respect of its deployment.

So what then can we say that KM 'is'? One of the earliest and most helpful definitions available to us was provided by Churchman in 1971, who stated that:

> To conceive of knowledge as a collection of information seems to rob the concept of all of its life. Knowledge resides in the user and not in the collection. It is how the user reacts to a collection of information that matters.
>
> (cited in Malhotra 1997:1)

Such a definition helps to focus our attention upon the two primary players in the KM dynamic: the human, most usually defined as the employee, and the way in which they interact with and use information. This is very much in alignment with the underpinning hypothesis of this text, which views IM as providing the necessary building blocks on the road to achieving an organisational culture that encourages KM. We can further contextualise this view by considering one of the opening statements of a 1998 KPMG research report, *The Power of Knowledge*, in which Parlby cautions us that: 'Knowledge Management is not an abstract proposition for the future ... it is a vital aspect of world-class management in today's business environment' (KPMG 1998a: ii). So KM is very firmly not a fad; what is new about it is that it represents 'a systematic and organised attempt to use knowledge within an organisation to transform its ability to store and use knowledge to improve performance' (KPMG 1998a: 5).

By marrying the views of Churchman and Parlby, outlined above, we are then able to ask ourselves what it is that we are advocating should be 'managed'. What can we realistically aspire to structure and make use of, in respect of something that is usually tacit, held in the repositories of employees' minds rather than filing cabinets or computer files? While it is impossible to arrive at a precise and all-encompassing list of what might be included, we should be aware that KM is usually found to refer to employees' perceptions, understanding and experience as they relate to functions and operations within and external to the organisation: 'Knowledge is a key resource in intelligent tasks such as decision-making, assessment, forecasting, design, planning diagnosis and analysis. It can be formal, systematic and explicitly recorded in repositories or it can be in people's minds as insight and intuition' (KPMG 1998a: 2).

Such a view offers considerable attractions to those political thinkers and senior-level public sector managers who are keen to move forward the emerging concept of the 'knowledge economy', focusing as it does on the increasing role of the 'knowledge worker', seen as an expensive and hitherto under-utilised organisational resource. In typical public service scenarios, we have only to consider the proportion of total budgets spent on staffing resources to understand that rich potential for change may be found through deploying and using human resources, at all operating levels, in different, more innovative and indeed possibly more intelligent ways.

The KPMG research report cited above provides some useful insights for anyone coming to the concept of KM for the first time. Particularly useful is the worked example of the data, information, knowledge transformation process outlined in Chapter 1, which puts forward a scenario based upon a railway timetable:

> A train timetable provides data (which must be interpreted to be useful).
> A platform announcement that the next train to the desired destination is leaving in five minutes provides information (having specific meaning in a given context).
> The passenger's realisation that the first train to reach the destination may not be the first to leave (since some are stopping trains and others express) depends on knowledge (it depends upon a more generally applicable model based on insight and experience).
> Data and information are vital resources, but it is the superior knowledge that produces the more effective decision and action.
>
> (KPMG 1998a: 2)

The challenge that few public service organisations have yet moved to address is how, in an organisational context, one can put strategies and structures in place to harness the power of this 'superior knowledge'. A key issue is that many have not yet successfully addressed issues of either data or information management, without which any move to apply KM is likely to be doomed from the outset.

Creating a KM-focused public service organisation

When considering sectors of the global economy where it is possible to iden-tify strong trends for the adoption of KM strategies, it is possible to map patterns which highlight the predominance of focus that exists in manage-ment consulting businesses, pharmaceutical companies and financial services sectors, particularly those which interact with their clients through call centre operations. It is important to ask, therefore, why such businesses have been early adopters of KM practice and to consider whether any of these identified factors might also have some commonality with public services. An analysis of KM-adopting organisations can lead us to make some generalisations; broadly speaking, they are

- working in industries where pressures for change, innovation and creativity are critical to success and business survival;
- building a relationship with a client and providing some element of tailor-made or value-added product or service upon which competitive advantage is built;
- likely to invest significant sums in staff training and development on an ongoing basis;
- information-intensive organisations with well-developed strategies for the identification and management of such resources;
- typically employing over a thousand people, often spread across diverse offices and sites.

When we examine these areas of commonality, there would appear to be a clear business case for the adoption of KM approaches. If we map this expe-rience against what might typically be found in a public service organisation, we can immediately recognise that in terms of size there are obvious syner-gies between KM adopting firms and the structures typically found in the public sector. The issue of size is not by any means an illusory one, for it is true to say that in organisations that might be classified as small and medium-sized enterprises (SMEs), typically employing no more than 750 people, the strength and impact of local knowledge networks, operating on a largely informal basis, are already likely to be largely effective. However, once a certain operating size and structural complexity have been reached, the influence and efficacy of informal mechanisms and avenues for informa-tion and knowledge exchange become diminished; at this point the importance and potential value of focusing on KM in a systematic manner should become apparent. Public service organisations are typically large in respect of numbers of employees, hierarchical in structure and often also complex in terms of geographical spread of offices and links to other func-tions of service provision or governance.

    If we also consider the fact that the public service operating environment is often dominated by an overarching 'political' change agenda, we can immediately recognise that there are some considerable synergies between those sectors identified as being early adopters of KM and public service operations. One of the key challenges facing public services in the twenty-first century is their readiness and ability to achieve appropriate levels of improvement through service innovation, and much, if not all, of this will have to be achieved within existing or even reduced financial operating parameters. To adopt a KM approach is to acknowledge that there is much to be gained from tapping into and utilising the knowledge-base and experience of the employee community in a structured and ongoing manner. However, as we discussed earlier, such an approach has been firmly rebutted by commentators such as Rutledge, on the basis that such a focus on the role of this group of 'stakeholders' is potentially dangerous, representing a dangerous dilution of – and possibly deviation from – a clearly articulated organisational focus on performance improvement (Rutledge 1997).

Whether the adoption of KM principles represents the proverbial 'threat' or 'opportunity' for public services depends in reality upon whether it is an overtly pragmatic or idealistic approach to the matter which is being employed. There are significant dangers inherent in adopting the language and rhetoric of KM in too reverential a manner for, after all, it is what is actually delivered, beyond the terminology, that actually matters. So while it is no doubt tempting to talk in terms of creating a knowledge-based and learning organisation, the fundamental question for any public service manager must be: what is this actually going to deliver? What are the tangibles associated with moving to different modes of working? Is what we are talking about realistic within present operating structures and cultures? If the answers to all or most of these questions seem negative, this does not mean that the blueprint for KM needs to be abandoned: rather, it needs to be thought through in an organisation-specific context.

The first step in moving towards achieving knowledge-driven improvements is for senior managers to recognise that their department or function is in the first instance an information-intensive operation. From recognition of this critical position, it should then be possible to introduce the notion that employees – typically representing more than 70 per cent of the operational cost of service provision – are in themselves information processors and users, and that their roles at almost all levels of the service will typically engage them in some aspect of knowledge generation and use. Information and knowledge, when articulated in this way, can then come to be seen as what they actually are. In the case of information, it is the fuel that drives the service machine; in the case of knowledge, it is opportunity for ongoing refinements and changes resulting in service evolution and appropriate innovation. To ignore the potential for harnessing and capitalising upon knowledge assets in a public service context is, therefore, to waste opportunities. It is also to neglect input from a key constituency group who may actually be closer to the end-user and their needs and responses to services than the strategists and their supporting data-gathering can ever hope to be.

Achieving a knowledge-based public service organisation: 'goodbye to all that'?

A problem when seeking to promote innovation and creativity in public services is that, in the twenty years since the Thatcher and Reagan reforms first came to the fore, many management approaches and methodologies developed in commercial sector scenarios have been deployed into this sector. This has usually been without any acknowledgement of the possible need for adaptation or any questioning of their underlying appropriateness to the distinct mission that public services must fulfil. To approach KM in this way is to invite failure, for although the rhetoric may be attractive – for example, as put forward in the UK government's 1998 White Paper on Competitiveness (Department for Trade and Industry 1998) – success will depend upon recognising that approaches must be tailor-made requirements of the organisation, and that essentially KM is rather more philosophy than distinct and prescriptive methodology.

So, given that KM is not a model or package that can be bought off the shelf and that even benchmarking activities with organisations in other sectors may provide nothing more than possible indicators for potential ways forward, how should a public sector manager seek to adopt and promote KM? First, there is a need to recognise that issues around knowledge and its management are part of a complex web which must be defined in an organisation-specific way. As Davenport and Prusak argue:

> Knowledge is neither data nor information, though it is related to both, and the differences between these terms are often a matter of degree ... Confusion about what data, information and knowledge are – how they differ, what those words *mean* – has resulted in enormous expenditures on technology initiatives that rarely deliver.
>
> (Davenport and Prusak 1998: 1)

Thus the first step towards achieving KM is to ask what it actually is, how it relates to other areas of operation and, fundamentally, what it is that you want to achieve. Just as with IM strategies, these issues of *definition* are critical to achieving both focus and success.

Because KM is about people and how they contribute to the organisation, issues of definition are something which need to be handled at a senior policy level, for ultimately a decision to adopt KM-based principles can lead to implications for recruitment, development, retention planning and service design itself. The public services that exist today, particularly as exemplified in developed economies, remain on the whole large, complex and hierarchi-

cally structured organisations, increasingly involved in client/contractor relationships with outsourced functions and third-party service providers.
However, despite the adoption of new structures and contract-based modes
of working, what remains at the heart of public service delivery is a lack of
focus upon *employees* as being the key to achieving innovation and success.
Rather, they are regarded, as they have been historically, as tools – exemplified by the commonly used term 'public servants' – rather than assets of
public service delivery.

Altering an historically entrenched mind-set which is arguably still shared
by a majority of politicians, understood by the public as the consumers of
services and indeed used as the *modus operandi* for a large majority of public
sector employees, requires considerable vision for anticipated outcomes and
considerable determination to overcome both internal and external resistance to change. At a senior political level, there is a fundamental need for
thought leadership in defining how we want twenty-first-century public
services to operate. Allied to this, of course, there needs to be a commensurate level of authority and commitment to deliver on the vision.

In respect of achieving KM in a public sector context, what would this
actually mean? If we consider the influential work of Nonaka and Takeuchi
and their analysis of key characteristics and critical success factors which
have driven forward the development of commercial and industrial enterprises in Japan, we have the opportunity to engage with an important and
useful perspective on the nature of knowledge in the organisational environment. Their model – developed, we must remember, with no reference to
public sector applications – presents a cyclical relationship: knowledge
creation leads to continuous innovation and results in competitive advantage
(Nonaka and Takeuchi 1995: 6). The commercial dynamic underpinning this
process is underlined by the use of examples drawn from the manufacturing
sector. For instance, the Matsushita company developed an automatic
bread-making machine by combining the expertise of three operational divisions to create one product. The product knowledge of three sets of workers,
previously making rice cookers, toasters and coffee makers, and food processors, was combined when the company amalgamated the three divisions and
set them new targets. Here, knowledge (in the form of experience and expertise), information (both technical and product-based) and a change in the
organisational environment led to innovation and the creation of a new
niche in the market.

Discussion of bread-makers, while interesting, has little that is obviously
in common with the provision and operation of services such as revenue
collection, benefits processing or education. And indeed, while the literature
around innovation-based commercial success in Japan is much in evidence, it
was only in the late 1990s that any of these methodologies became in any
way influential in the design and delivery of public services (Brockman 1997).
Yet if we consider the processes that are being discussed here, it is possible to

consider whether they are in reality so very different from those which have impacted upon converged or reconstituted public sector organisations such as the Centrelink example discussed in Chapter 3, where reconfigured teams of people have been drawn together into new operating structures. A key difference perhaps is that those involved in developing bread-makers appeared to have innovation at the core of their rationale for change, while in public sector scenarios, rationalisation and efficiency appear to be the dominant drivers of change. Yet this is a perception that demands to be challenged, for it serves to focus on the key conceptual questions that those involved in moving forward the public service agenda at a policy level must ask:

• Do we want a less expensive way of delivering public services?
• Do we want qualitatively *different* public services?

Consideration of these two questions should not be seen as mutually exclusive. What is rather more important is the order in which they are taken: if it is questions of cost that are allowed to predominate above issues of innovation, then the likelihood is that less than satisfactory outcomes will result.

How, then, can concepts of KM be usefully harnessed within a strategy for change and innovation in the public sector, one that may actually result in static or reduced costs but in alignment with a goal of improved services? A crucial step is in moving to understand what knowledge is, moving it from an admittedly abstract base to something which can be grounded in applied contexts. Again, the work of Nonaka and Takeuchi is useful in constructing an approach that lends itself to analysing knowledge processes, something they define as *tacit* and *explicit* classifications (Nonaka and Takeuchi 1995: 6).

This tacit/explicit definition of how organisations could usefully seek to consider their approach to identifying and managing knowledge has been much discussed by theorists and practitioners. Snowden argues that one way to understand the relationship between tacit and explicit knowledge is to look at ways in which they are shared and stored. In his opinion, explicit knowledge is:

> reusable in a consistent and repeatable manner. It may be stored in a written procedure, in a manual or as a process in a computer system … it exists as a physical or virtual entity that can be measured, identified and distributed. It is explicit.
>
> (cited in Rock 1998: 10)

It is in respect of this definition of knowledge that public sector organisations can be said to have traditionally focused their interests and activities. Adherence to explicitly stated procedures which have evolved from practice-based scenarios is, for most organisations that operate within the remit of the public sector, where their interaction with issues of knowledge often begins and usually ends.

However, if we consider the other side of the model, which is concerned with *tacit* knowledge, we find an approach that is unfamiliar to very many organisations, and not simply those operating within the public sector. This is an area which is concerned with extracting value from and giving some structure to

> something we know, possibly without the ability to explain. ... Human beings are the storage medium of tacit knowledge. When the storage medium is an individual then it is vulnerable to loss; where it is stored in a community the vulnerability is reduced, the ability to reuse is enhanced.
>
> (Rock 1998: 10)

The focus here is therefore very much upon an organisation's people and their relationship with one another, maximising the value that accrues from encouraging people to work together, collaboratively in an informal sense or perhaps in more structured team or project-based modes. Such an approach demands that organisational structures and resulting cultures be examined and understood by those who seek to achieve innovative approaches to service delivery. In order to succeed, there must be an acknowledgement that

> the sharing of tacit knowledge among multiple individuals with different backgrounds, perspectives, and motivations becomes the critical step for organisational knowledge creation to take place. The individual's emotions, feelings and mental models have to be shared to build mutual trust.
>
> (Nonaka and Takeuchi 1995: 85)

The concepts introduced here of knowledge sharing and the cross-boundary working that this implies are generally held to represent the foundations of achieving an organisation that positively manages innovation and creativity. For Nonaka and Takeuchi, the movement from the conceptual to the applied, in achieving this type of knowledge-utilising organisation, is reliant upon what they describe as the 'middle-up-down' management process (Nonaka and Takeuchi 1995: 150). They argue that the creation (and ultimately successful exploitation) of organisational knowledge is dependent on the close interaction of the individuals directly employed within the organisation. To broaden the perspective through the public sector paradigm, this should also include those working in closely related departments or agencies. Middle managers, in contact with both top management and front-line staff, are, in this scenario, in a unique position to facilitate and promote a culture of interaction and knowledge-sharing in a way that traditional and still dominant hierarchical structures cannot.

Seeking to harness and manage the value of organisational knowledge can, therefore, be said to represent a considerable challenge to accepted notions of how public services should be structured and operate. As has been previously argued, despite the considerable reforms undertaken during the 1980s, the dominant issues appeared to be those that focused upon cost reduction, together with the importation of practices from the commercial sector regarded as offering the opportunity for redefining what was sometimes disparagingly referred to as a public service 'ethos'. Issues around public sector deployment of KM invite comparison with these 1980s trends of politicians advocating direct adoption of emerging tools and techniques from other sectors, and do give reasonable grounds for concern. If, as we have seen, what KM should primarily be focusing upon is the creation and maintenance of a knowledge-rich, open and creative operating culture, how can the public service structures that have developed in the last two decades be adapted or restructured to achieve the greatest benefits? Is it, in fact, realistic to think in terms of 'relaunching' the concept of public service organisational structure and operating culture? Can KM be imposed in much the same way as contracting-out and service-level agreements were in the 1980s?

The answer to these three questions is a qualified 'maybe', but it is a response that must be couched in terms which acknowledge that KM has rather more to do with evolution than revolution. In reality, public services are usually far removed from the moribund, backward-looking, change-resisting structures that are often portrayed in the media. Modern public services, such as those evident in the USA, the UK, Canada and Australia, are built upon a complex operational web, dependent upon a network of internal and external relationships for their ability to function. They are typically structured to manage these relationships in a hierarchical and contract-driven manner which can serve to reduce or possibly destroy any opportunities for developing an open and knowledge-driven operating culture. It is unrealistic to argue that, however keen politicians may be, public services can or would necessarily want to say goodbye to the constraints of present structures. Even so, discussions around issues of creating a knowledge leveraging culture can encourage examination of current practice and consideration of how it can profitably be developed, bearing in mind that for almost all national governments there is some notion of an ongoing change agenda in respect of public sector structures and rationale.

Creating a KM culture: the problems of outsourcing and enabling

This chapter has highlighted the critical issues of promoting knowledge sharing and the breaking down of traditional operating barriers as key factors in moving towards the achievement of a knowledge-driven organisational culture. However, during the decade of change that characterised the 1980s, a new notion of public services developed, one which saw all tiers of government being encouraged – and in some instances legislated – to view and structure themselves as 'enablers' rather than direct 'providers' of services to the public. In the United Kingdom, which was in the vanguard of pressing forward change in this area, the first focus of activity was upon the way in which local authorities were structured to provide services under their remit. Some of the impetus for this change agenda was summarised by Sparke, who argued that

> much store is set by politicians on the number of persons employed by Local Authorities. Head counts have therefore become a consideration, secondary only to cash expenditure, informing the Government's public sector borrowing requirement and the standard spending assessments used to determine how much centrally allocated money is passed to Local Authorities ... It needs to be recognised that externalisation immediately reduces the numbers of public sector employees and any counterbalancing increase in private sector employment will not affect the kudos attached to the former.
>
> (Sparke 1994: 11)

This somewhat crude accounting method presents a key structural challenge for those focused upon developing a more creative and innovative public service ethos. The model developed in the UK, which was drawn to some extent upon practice in the United States and New Zealand, has left a legacy of public service structures where it is possible to plot the potential barriers in the contractual and largely rigid relationships created in a move towards enabler-focused structures. This model is repeated in very many nations.

In the commercial sector, particularly in manufacturing industries, this type of relationship has often been commonplace in the linkages between a major contractor and its subcontracting suppliers of components. Consider the hugely competitive automotive engineering manufacture sector, which is to a great extent dependent for success upon the ability to be innovative and flexible in terms of the product design/manufacture life cycle. From a base of the 1960s and 1970s, it is possible to plot many of the barriers that public service re-engineering of the 1980s has created in achieving a culture of innovation.

Global economic crises of the 1970s, particularly the instability arising from what is now usually referred to as the 'oil crisis', had a profound and lasting effect upon the way in which major European and North American motor manufacturers were structured to do business. A continued post-war period of economic growth had led to considerable complacency, particularly in respect to investment in new product design and, still more critically, to the fostering of relationships with subcontractors, on whom multinational corporations such as General Motors and Ford remained dependent for the supply of key product components. This approach was in marked contrast with the modes of operation adopted by their emerging Japanese competitors, for whom innovation was held to be an organisation-wide responsibility and for whom collaboration with subcontractors was the norm, rather than the traditional client/provider model prevalent in the West. Much has been written about the philosophies adopted by Japanese companies as they demonstrated that their participative and collaborative approach to business resulted in sustained growth for a period of almost two decades. With respect to the public sector operating scenario, however, there is a great deal emerging from this particular example that lends itself to consideration in respect of the implementation of KM approaches. Primarily, of course, the synergies lie in considering how operating structures can be created to promote development and improvement.

In a public sector context, possibly the greatest barriers to KM arise from the cultures and contracts which serve to impede rather than support the collaborative and improvement-focused culture identified as being pivotal in moving forward large swathes of Japanese industry. To consider one relatively small-scale example of the barriers to information and knowledge-sharing that have been erected in the structuring of modern public services, it is useful to consider the example of a small public library service in the United Kingdom. Given the relatively non-controversial nature of this sector and the fact that it might be expected that library services at least would be structured in such a way as to focus upon prioritising use of information, the lessons emerging can be magnified many times over in larger-scale restructuring, such as the Centrelink initiative previously discussed.

Our example concerns a small local authority within London. Its approach to the provision of public library services was to create what it referred to as a 'client–contractor split'. Without actually externalising the provision of library services (it was established that there was not a viable external provider pool) the council effectively 'split' its library establishment into two operating units: the 'contractors' – the actual service points – and the 'clients', represented by a nucleus of management and monitoring staff whose duty was to set specifications on behalf of the council and to monitor and reward or penalise achievements measured against defined criteria. While such an approach may be characterised as innovative, one must surely ask the question: to what extent was it likely to engender best use of staff and ongoing enhancement of services?

The resulting library service, although possibly qualitatively no worse than any other in the UK, was one where relationships between colleagues could be argued to have been distorted by the imposition of barriers to collaboration. Within what remained, titularly at least, the same service, colleagues became at extremes the monitors and the monitored; in view of this, it can be hardly surprising to learn anecdotally that previously good relationships across service points were to some extent replaced by suspicion and reluctance to share and exchange ideas and perceptions. And if one was to attempt to parachute a vision of KM into this scenario and culture, then the question would be: would it be able to penetrate the culture that had grown up around the operating structure? The answer, of course, would depend very much upon where KM had been 'parachuted' from, and its authority to move away from an avowedly 'split' mode of operation.

Of course, such an example is of very restricted size and influence. Nonetheless, it provides an important means of illustrating the cultural barriers to KM that have accrued over the decades when purely contractual relationships have emerged as the dominant mode in redefining public service operating structures. Just as we saw that the success of Japanese motor manufacturers was dependent, at least in some part, upon the emphasis on encouraging innovation among internally employed personnel and on dialogue and appropriate collaboration with external suppliers, so we can see that, for KM to take hold and flourish in a public sector scenario, there is a clear need for relationships and channels of communication within and across departmental or functional structures to be understood in respect of a clearly delineated KM agenda.

To consider on a rather larger scale the barriers that modern public sector structures can present to knowledge sharing and creativity, we should look once more at the example of Centrelink. The rationale for this multi-function collapsing of numerous government services under one operating umbrella was undoubtedly to bring about a structure that facilitated considerable contracting out of services to external providers. This was particularly so in respect of employment services. Thus, very many of the traditional employment counselling and placement services previously provided directly by the Commonwealth Government were contracted out to external providers. Now, it is true to say that there exists a relatively mature employment services industry which has proved itself undoubtedly capable of taking on and to some extent repackaging employment 'products' in a manner which allows politicians to point to a reduced public sector payroll. However, questions must remain around the extent to which the nature of the contractual relationship created has actually served to starve Centrelink of much valuable operational and strategic knowledge. By this we mean that the knowledge-base of the Australian government, in respect of employment services, is based primarily upon statistical data provided by its contractors, and this must be viewed in light of the fact that many of these commercially geared organisations are effectively in competition with one another. Centrelink itself undertakes to provide services directly only to clients who are difficult to place, such as those in geographically remote areas or those who are perhaps disabled in some way; as such, it can be said to have only a very partial perspective upon which to plan for the development of employment services on a national scale.

Now it should be noted that this focus on Centrelink is intended in no way to diminish either the scale of the undertaking represented or the innovative approaches that underpin it. Rather, what are being highlighted here are the problems that operational structures and resulting cultures can have upon the achievement of an evolving and knowledge-driven mode of service delivery. What we have seen in the example of a small UK public library service and in the far larger Australian example is that the trends of two decades, which have moved public services in the direction of adopting primarily an enabling focus, have served in our present context to present significant barriers to ongoing and informed innovation in the public service arena.

Knowledge management and people: plotting a way forward

Given that the adoption of KM strategies is largely contingent upon achieving an open and innovation-friendly operating culture, one must question the extent to which the practices and philosophies that dominate modern modes of operation in this sector present insuperable barriers to achieving KM-driven change. Certainly, as we have discussed, the adoption of client/contractor and outsourcing relationships at all levels of government has served to erect potentially significant barriers to both sharing and learning. However, this is not to suggest that at least some strands of KM may prove capable of adaptation for deployment across this diverse environment.

If we consider once more the premise underpinning this book – an explicit linkage between the management of information and knowledge – it is immediately apparent that a primary focus upon managing information assets is likely to result in some shift of operating culture. Where there is a determination at senior level to ensure that information is used in an efficient and effective manner, then this cannot but impact upon the relationships within and between distinct operating units. An organisational culture that understands its information needs and priorities and which properly focuses its ICT applications upon supporting clearly articulated processes and goals is one where, at a mature stage of implementation, at least some evidence of the benefits accruing from sharing information is likely to be acknowledged. Without addressing this stage of IM and building good practice into emerging public service structures, the likelihood of successfully moving forward issues of KM is remote.

A precursor of KM which received a good deal of interest from both politicians and senior managers in the early 1990s was the concept of 'empowerment', a much used and (lately) frequently derided term which has much synergy with certain elements of KM. Empowering employees, devolving authority to the 'front line', these and much more became mantras of management gurus and consultants alike. However, the reality has often proved to be less than satisfactory, with public sector attempts to embed empowerment approaches in applied contexts usually reported as having failed due to widespread resistance to notions of delegating authority and responsibility. Conversely, the other side of empowerment theory, which stresses the importance of encouraging 'up–down' channels of communication and exchange of ideas, has also failed to bring significant returns in public sector environments; once again the structure and cultures of these organisations presents the greatest barriers to encouraging sharing of ideas and observations.

Historically, the longest-established methodology for encouraging employee participation in the organisational innovation process has been through the medium of employee suggestion schemes, developed to various degrees in organisations drawn from all sectors, and with a relatively low profile in discussions around the shaping of employee behaviour and motivation patterns. Suggestion schemes have, in the era of KM, largely fallen from grace; they are perceived as old-fashioned and rigid in outlook, yet it can be argued that there is much that can be learned in developing effective KM strategies by considering the way in which suggestion scheme approaches developed. To take, for example, a view put forward in 1957 by the British Productivity Council:

> Every organisation has its own particular feel or atmosphere – happy or unhappy, optimistic or defeated, lively or apathetic. No activity remains unaffected by it, least of all a suggestion scheme, dependent as it must be on cooperation and trust. Suggestion schemes have a very useful part to play in fostering good relations, but they will not by themselves provide a basis for them. And they are no panacea for bad relations.
>
> (British Productivity Council 1957: 2)

Perhaps the central flaw in respect of suggestion schemes – and one which KM attempts to address – is the fact that the management of knowledge is not purely seeking to tap into new ideas and concepts. Rather, it is about capitalising upon that which is largely tacit – the ideas, certainly, but also the observations, perceptions and experiences of the human resource base. Moving towards the achievement of KM is about making linkages between various pieces of tacit knowledge and also with explicit, tangible and ongoing projects and concepts. While the suggestion scheme methodology is reliant upon the explicit articulation of innovation, KM is rather more about supporting the emergence of innovation and creativity and decisions relating to these processes. Nonetheless, the need for co-operation and trust is identical in respect of both approaches, and presents potentially the greatest challenge to the cause of KM.

Knowledge management and technology

In Chapter 6 we will consider in some detail the ICT applications that can support both IM and KM, but it is important in the context of this discussion of issues around knowledge to consider the ways in which technological developments serve to highlight the degree of missed opportunities in extracting maximum value from the interactions of employees. For example, it is now common for a great deal of intra- and inter-office communications to take place via electronic mail, not only opening up opportunities for increasing the speed of communications, but also making wide-scale sharing of this communication far more practical. However, commonly this takes place in an unstructured and ad hoc manner, with little thought being given to the possible benefits that might accrue from having a more thought-out approach to the destinations of even informal observational materials. In recent years, software applications, often referred to as 'intelligent agents', have been held out as offering an automated approach to embedding this structure into electronic channels of communication which may be potentially knowledge-rich. Indeed, a number of public sector organisations have already expressed interest in purchasing such 'solutions'. Yet this is to presume that the knowledge 'products' that accrue from such applications have both the focus and the commitment of those operating within the organisation.

Far more important than early investment in intelligent agent software and so-called expert systems for any organisation, particularly where resources are scarce, is to consider how a knowledge-creating, knowledge-sharing culture can be developed. Then, and only then, can it profit from the deployment of sophisticated enabling software. Fundamentally, what this requires is that recruitment and development activity focuses upon investing in the human resource base of the organisation in ways which promote the embedding of KM philosophies within the normal operating environment. So, while it may appear deeply old-fashioned, the appropriate and successful deployment of software such as intelligent agents is ultimately reliant upon educating and monitoring the workforce in respect of good practice. This, combined, with a realisation that quantifiable returns are unlikely to be immediate, presents significant challenges in respect of moving forward the public sector case for KM.

The employee and KM

Probably the best-developed use of KM strategies in an organisational context is to be found in the practices of the major globally operating management consultancies, where the essence of their continued success is reliant upon retaining and building the client base through utilisation of internally and externally held information and knowledge assets. In recent years, the emphasis upon KM has grown considerably, with many practices appointing senior-level 'chief knowledge officers' or equivalent, whose remit is to ensure that the organisation is utilising and maximising the value of the explicit and tacit knowledge holdings of its employees. The approaches adopted in these large, diverse and hugely profitable organisations offer some pointers as to the challenges and opportunities that face public sector operating contexts if they are to move towards the successful adoption of KM.

The appointment of chief knowledge officers, at least some of whom have built their earlier careers in the area of human resource management, has served to focus aspects of ongoing employee training, development and appraisal processes on issues of KM. Specifically, there has been a recognition that much of the work of consultancies, not unlike large swathes of public service activity, is run on a project basis, where personnel may work together as a multi-disciplinary team for a period of time, sometimes running into a number of years, and that during the life cycle of projects experience and tacit knowledge is gained which hitherto had been unrecorded. Thus, at the end of a project or upon the departure of a member of staff, much that might potentially be of use to other projects or groups would be effectively lost.

To counterbalance the effects of knowledge loss and leakage, education has been identified as the first stage in promoting the development of a knowledge-aware operating culture. Typically, induction and ongoing staff development programmes incorporate sessions on the recognition of what knowledge is, and the contribution, through the use of worked examples, that it may potentially make to the overall success of the organisation. Critically, training and ongoing development in this area are not targeted only at 'key' groups of employees, for in a KM-driven culture *all* employees are potentially capable of making a contribution. Of course, to take this approach and seek to transfer it into a public sector scenario would require considerable commitment and authority on the part of the senior manager(s), for training programmes that may often involve thousands of employees can represent a major investment of resources. Also, experience has demonstrated that such blanket approaches to training in support of an 'initiative' can result in nothing more than short-term benefits and longer-term cynicism.

The approach adopted in the consultancy sector to counteract the dangers of short-termism accruing from investment in training has been twofold. In the first instance, KM education and development is not normally treated as a 'one-off' activity, that once completed is never revisited. Rather, what commonly happens is that issues of KM, which as we have seen do in practice interact with a great many other strands of organisational management practice, are incorporated into the organisation-wide portfolio of training opportunities. Similarly, a further strand of embedding KM into the operating culture has been the inclusion of aspects of individual performance in relation to knowledge sharing and use in the performance appraisal process. Emerging indicators of evaluation in this area have typically been around monitoring the relationships that individual employees build with other practice areas and, increasingly, the usage patterns of personally created and maintained web pages that form part of the company-wide Intranet.

In a public sector scenario it is possible to build many arguments around why such an approach to KM would be impossible to take forward successfully. However, consider first the issue around ongoing training and development: public sector organisations do invest in staff development, but typically they do so on a stovepipe approach, with little underpinning coherence to the range of opportunities offered. The success evident in the consultancy sector, resulting from KM training, comes from an operating stance in which knowledge is generally a clearly articulated and understood business asset, and has no tensions or difficulties in co-existing alongside other business priorities. To achieve this type of approach would not necessarily require public sector organisations to increase their spend on training, but rather to evaluate existing provision in respect of what type of culture it is helping to create. Such an holistic view of the potential for engendering a knowledge-based culture is one that no major public sector organisation has yet adopted.

So what, then, of the use of performance appraisal opportunities to drive forward and embed approaches to KM? In the consultancy sector, of course, there is widespread adoption of salary enhancement in relation to evaluation of performance, something which typically in public service organisations is only evident among more senior employees. However, this is not to discount the potentially powerful and beneficial influence that performance measurement may have upon behaviour, even if this is not always linked to financial incentives. Assuming that relevant evaluation criteria were developed, there is little reason to prevent contribution to KM activities being monitored routinely, with the resultant behaviour profiles of employees being fed into an ongoing review of development and training opportunities.

At the close of this consideration of KM, it is undoubtedly appropriate to question whether there is a likelihood that this approach can realistically achieve widespread adoption in public service organisations. As yet there are few examples of KM activity in the public sector, yet, perhaps paradoxically, the issue of knowledge is increasingly espoused by politicians as holding the key to ensuring ongoing economic success. What is now needed is for a major national government to look inward upon its own operating structures and to assess how the adoption of KM might result in the achievement of qualitatively better services, stemming from a more intelligent use of employees. However, to do this will require that hard and searching questions are asked around the way in which the public sector is structured as it enters the twenty-first century, and the barriers that certain approaches may present to moving forward the goal of achieving a knowledge-efficient operating culture. If such questions remain unasked, and if there remains no clear vision of what KM is actually expected to deliver, then there is every reason to anticipate that the impact upon public service design and operation will be no more than peripheral.

Chapter 5

Managing information, ideas and solutions

A focus on the employee

If the achievement of effective information and knowledge management (IKM) can be said to be dependent upon one factor above any other, it must surely be the importance that is attached to maximising the value of organisational input made by employees. In previous chapters the discussion of issues around IKM has focused upon important concepts that are contained within and interact with these linked management disciplines. However, somewhat paradoxically, it is the pivotal role that the public sector employee, working at all levels and across all functions of public service, can play in the achievement of a dynamic information and knowledge generating and utilising organisational structure, that remains the least understood and least practised route to achieving public sector change and improvement agendas. As Drucker argues: 'All organizations now say routinely, "People are our greatest asset." Yet few practice what they preach, let alone truly believe it' (Drucker 1992: 8).

Typically, as we have previously discussed, public services are human resource-intensive structures, even when, for political and accounting purposes, at least some employees may notionally be employed only indirectly by public service authorities. Importantly, external perceptions attached to the public sector employee can vary widely, with civil service and public sector posts remaining high-status and comparatively high-income career choices most commonly in newly emerging economies, such as South Africa and the countries of Eastern Europe. However, since the early 1980s there has been a marked decline in the status and relative attractiveness of public service careers in the United Kingdom, North America and Australia. Importantly, too, it appears increasingly rare for cross-fertilisation between public sector and private sector organisations to take place, through evidence of recruitment practices spanning both domains, particularly at a middle and senior management level. Exceptions to this pattern are to be found in nations such as France, which has retained a proportionately high degree of public sector ownership of the industrial and utilities base of the nation, and where there remains a tradition of ready interchange between the 'commercial' interests of the government and the more clearly defined public service element.

However, despite there being evidence of some exceptions, the majority of public service employees enter the twenty-first century in a markedly different position from that of even twenty years ago. The change agenda is, for a majority, a constant feature of working life, as true at the highest echelons of government departments and service structures as it is at the point of service delivery. Alongside this must be set, of course, the impact that diminishing employment status and comparable remuneration has undoubtedly had upon recruitment, retention and levels of morale. The focus of this chapter is therefore to consider how, within public sector constraints and change pressures, the management of information, ideas and solutions can be used to build a more positive operational culture, one which may serve as a powerful catalyst for rebuilding and redefining what it means to be employed within modern public services.

It is interesting, when reflecting on the evolution of concepts around IKM, to consider the way in which the focus upon the management of people has shifted over time. Until the 1980s, academic study and professional practice most often referred to the notion of 'personnel management'; more recently, and influenced considerably by issues around quality management, it has been widely referred to as 'human resource management'. However, increasingly a new term is evolving, one which has considerable affinity with KM, and that is an approach that advocates the management of 'human capital'. As defined by Friedman *et al.* such an approach is crucial to the achievement of future organisational success:

> In order to value people, companies must move beyond the notion of human resources and toward the notion of human capital. The very term *resource* (from the Latin *resurgere*, to rise again) implies an available supply that can be drawn upon when needed. ... But are people really a 'resource' in this sense? Or are they more like a form of *capital* – something that gains or loses value depending upon how much we invest in it?
>
> (Friedman *et al.* 1998: 2)

The answer to the questions posed above, in the context of achieving IKM, must surely be that the most appropriate way to build a culture that supports and nurtures the creation and use of information and knowledge is to look positively at the notion of 'human capital'. Fundamentally, as we stated in the opening chapter, public service organisations, like commercial sector businesses such as financial services, are information- and knowledge-intensive operations. A key difference between the two sectors, however, is perhaps the relative importance that they place upon investing in their people as assets of, rather than costs to, the organisation. Typically, despite some rhetoric around the importance and value of public sector employees, there is little evidence as yet to point to any sustained examples of adoption of a human capital approach to the management of employees. The purpose of this chapter is therefore, in substantial part, to consider strategies for moving forward the achievement of public sector cultures where IKM can thrive and evolve, through the adoption and adaptation of employee management approaches that focus upon issues of developing and involving this form of 'capital' in a far more planned and systematic manner than previously considered.

Focus on the employee: the challenges ahead

As soon as one considers the terminology prevalent when discussing public service employees, where there is much use of the word 'servant' and military terminology such as 'government officer', an immediate tension becomes apparent between the aspirations of the human capital approach to management and the operating cultures that have evolved. A 'public servant' has traditionally been regarded as just that, someone who is delivering, at various levels of seniority, someone else's agenda, just as an 'officer' is duty bound to be a conduit of higher-level orders. Even in an age of outsourced and agency-based working, much of this historically redolent language – and indeed associated hierarchy-bound attitudes – remains prevalent in the public service domain. So what scale of cultural change is needed to make IKM work likely to succeed or fail, on the basis of the ability and willingness of public services to adopt aspects of a human capital approach to employment practice?

If we consider the perspective put forward in the KPMG report on 'the power of knowledge', we can immediately identify some of the possible challenges ahead:

> Moving to a culture that values and encourages innovation, openness, teamwork and knowledge sharing requires leadership and possibly changes in relationships, organisational structures and office environment. Management should consider what they need to do to start and sustain this change and, in particular on their roles as examples to staff. Thorough and sustainable cultural change takes time, but some useful initiatives can be taken quite quickly. For example, the creation of a time and place where staff can meet to discuss their ideas and experiences that is clearly viewed by senior management as an investment rather than a cost, can produce a tangible outcome and also have deeper symbolic effect.
>
> (KPMG 1998a: 9)

Such a view is somewhat removed from the model of public service delivery that has, despite much change pressure, retained a largely hierarchical and predominantly non-participative mode of operation. So to what extent is it realistic to posit an approach to both structure and management, that is culturally alien, or at the very least unfamiliar, to a majority of public services? Within the context not only of moving forward the cause of IKM but also of taking as a broader perspective the achievement of more effective, cost-efficient modes of public service delivery, the development of new modes of working and of more dynamic and engaging workplace environments would appear to offer the most realistic opportunity for enacting positive change agenda.

Thus, whether the discussion at a strategic level is around issues of 'human capital' or 'information and knowledge management', the focus on the employee must be a critical component. However, there are considerable dangers that the required degree of employee focus will never truly happen, that rhetorical approaches to these issues will take place at a political and senior level without ever actually engaging with the vast proportion of the human assets that typically comprise the organisation. As Fenton-O'Creevy astutely observes: 'The challenge for most organisations is not to decide whether to involve employees more but to simply get on and do it!' (Fenton-O'Creevy 1995: 51). This points to a central issue afflicting – and this word is used advisedly – a significant proportion of global public sector structures: the lack of clear focus upon precisely what change strategies are actually expected to deliver and how the employees fit into a new construction of public services. The result of this is that the employee resource base, far from having a sense of involvement in and willingness to contribute to the achievement of politically driven change agenda, is typically left feeling disenfranchised and disenchanted. This is a situation which no amount of allusion to 'knowledge-based' services or 'human-capital' focused organisations can hope to overcome, unless there is a clearly understood commitment on the part of policy- and strategy-makers to actually make it happen: in effect, 'to get on and do it' (Fenton-O'Creevy 1995: 51).

How to 'get on and do it': applying aspects of a linked human capital/IKM approach to public service design and delivery

If one accepts the premise that the creation of successful information- and knowledge-focused organisational cultures is essential in developing a new model of public service administration and service delivery, then the question must be asked: how can the rhetoric be moved forward into tangible change? No neat, bolt-on solutions can be applied to something which is so fundamental, but, as Friedman *et al.* (1998) advocate, there are perhaps five distinct stages that can usefully be used as a framework for moving forward effective changes in organisational culture.

Classification

If we take this as a crucial first stage in working towards building an IKM-friendly organisation, what is actually being advocated is that senior managers clearly articulate the goals of their service or function, and then relate them to the impact that they will have on the 'human capital' employed within the organisation. If we consider the example of employment services, elements of which we have already discussed in relation to the Australian example of Centrelink and currently much discussed in the UK and the United States, it is possible to map two generalisable goals or missions emerging in the late 1990s. The first is a clearly articulated intention to reduce and work towards the elimination of what is often referred to as the 'benefit culture'. The second, which is clearly linked to the first, is to move towards a much more pro-active approach to employment counselling, whereby 'clients' are required to attend interviews with employment service personnel on a far more regular basis than ever before, with failure to comply resulting in the withdrawal of benefit entitlement in some cases.

Such developments represent major cultural changes in themselves, changes which clearly have implications not only for various client groups, but also for those who are charged with ensuring that new systems and processes work effectively. Typically, however, roll-out of new policies is based upon a fairly narrow hierarchy of input which might see the following pattern emerge:

1   Advisory report prepared for politicians and senior civil servants based upon analysis of current practice, measured against international practice in similar public sector services and possibly also some benchmarking against practice in other sectors.
2   Feasibility studies prepared by external parties or senior civil servants, typically putting forward, where appropriate, cost/benefit analyses of a range of different approaches for ministerial consideration.
3   Increasingly, at the decision-making stage, some input may be sought from other interested agencies and also, on occasion, from citizens themselves via opinion-gathering mechanisms such as opinion surveys and focus groups.
4   Changes are framed in alignment with selected inputs from the above, which critically marry with the manifesto and direction of those politicians in positions of authority.

Analysis of these four stages begs the question, of course, of whether and indeed how existing information and knowledge assets, particularly the tacit knowledge of employees, fits into this pattern of policy and service development. As we have previously discussed with regard to Centrelink in Australia, the question of the employee as an asset, phrased in respect of something akin to the human capital approach, is a concept that appears largely alien in this *definition* and *classification* stage of actually bringing about change. Whether this is because, as Fenton-O'Creevy argues, there is a view prevalent that believes that 'employee involvement does not work – there is a lack of self discipline and strong leadership is necessary' or whether it is a less principled but nonetheless worrying ignorance of the employee as being anything other than 'a pair of hands', the results are the same: frequently the creation of low morale at the operational level and, of course, failure to utilise a key resource of the organisation, with all the waste that implies (Fenton-O'Creevy 1995: 32).

Thus if we are seeking to develop a 'checklist' of good practice in how to approach the reengineering of public services, we must first ensure that, when new policies and strategies are being developed, the change agenda includes scope to involve and utilise, on an ongoing basis, the knowledge base and experience of employees at all operating levels. Such a development, which should be regarded as proper utilisation of an existing resource rather than as a time-consuming *cost*, is not intended to impede the progress of change, but rather to ensure that changes that are actioned are more likely to succeed, because they have been informed by the experience of the employee base.

In the 1980s considerable discussion emerged from the Quality Management fields in relation to the role of the employee in achieving the much desired outcomes of 'continuous improvement'. In relation to this there was discernible organisational activity, particularly in respect of the creation of groupings such as Quality Circles. However, although such approaches have undoubtedly fed into the emerging field of information and knowledge management, what they fundamentally failed to achieve was a sustained focus upon the employee as an asset. When setting out our criteria for successfully moving forward public services, what we mean by focusing upon *classification* as an essential component in achieving successful outcomes is that the importance of utilising employees' information and knowledge base must be clearly articulated from the outset, and then actioned in respect of achieving maximum beneficial input to the development of effective strategies, goals and operating culture. Had such an approach been evident in respect of changes made in employment service reform, then, for example, issues like those arising from the increase in the number of formal interviews required between the client and the service might have been successfully addressed prior to implementation, with associated benefits accruing around the use of the employment service resource base.

Assessment

Having embedded the notion that maximising the value of employees to achieving successful change is reliant upon articulating this at the outset and building it into ongoing systems of service design and review, the question then becomes: how do you actually do this, and how do you evaluate success or failure? Accounting approaches based upon costs and benefits have never represented a precise mathematical formula; rather, they are an indicator upon which decisions can be supported, and in respect of assessing the likely impact of a more creative use of employee assets, this is likely to be the most useful means of framing an argument supporting developments that drive forward the creation of a more open information and knowledge-aware culture.

Employees who have no perception of themselves as 'assets' and no tradition of workplace practice encouraging the sharing of information and ideas are unlikely to suddenly adopt a set of behaviours that drive forward the development of such practices. As we have already discussed, there is much evidence of rhetoric at both a political and senior management level concerning what it means to be a public sector employee. Equally, however, there is scarcely any evidence of a properly thought-through strategy for ensuring not only that employees are able, outside the scope of normal work tasks, to make a contribution to the way in which their organisation works, but also that they understand this to be an important part of their working life.

If the first and critical phase, that of classification, is adhered to, then it should be self-evident that employees need to be supported and educated in learning new work-related behaviours. If the intention is ultimately to create an information and knowledge creating and utilising culture, then there must first be an assessment of exactly how the organisation currently performs. For example, if employment service personnel conducting client interviews simply record input while resulting data is not shared, compared, analysed and discussed with other colleagues, what changes need to be made to ensure that greater value is added to the procedure? Certainly there are resource implications: employees may need training beyond the need for expertise at the client-interface stage, and it may be that evaluation and analysis techniques, combined with mechanisms for exchanging perceptions and views with colleagues on a regular basis, could actually result in a more effective and efficient service.

There are, of course, clear additional costs associated with this approach and these must be assessed, as staff development and staff time are both potentially resource-intensive. Yet balanced against this – and this is where the imprecision of any cost/benefit methodology becomes immediately apparent – should be the likely benefits and potential savings that are considered likely to accrue from making greater use of costly human capital. Tangible savings are most likely to emerge from reductions in wasteful and duplicated operations which may be invisible to those charged with overall service design but are a fact of everyday life for front-line employees. Parallel to this, but even more difficult to quantify in accounting terms, is the likelihood that greater engagement by employees at all levels and the engendering of a culture where exchanging ideas and observations becomes the norm will result in a far more flexible and responsive service organisation. As Haak and Lekanne Deprez observe: 'the success of knowledge intensive organizations will ultimately depend on the speed of the organizational learning, the ability to effectively mobilize their knowledge and people base and turn it into value' (Haak and Lekanne Deprez 1998: 1).

Thus the assessment phase in building an IKM-focused public sector organisation is a critical one. It requires that, having acknowledged that employees are a critical component in creating and driving forward both the change agenda and a supportive operational environment, there must then be a clearly articulated assessment of what this actually means in practice. Making assumptions around automatic employee willingness, understanding and participation are not steps that are likely to result in success. Rather, what is needed is a clear understanding of current operations and the way in which employees work within these existing systems and structures. Then, the vision or mission of the service must be considered in the light of informed understanding of present practice, by means of some assessment of the gap between observed reality and the steps needed to bring about improved services. Therefore, for example, if it is decided at a policy level to increase the number and frequency of client interviews by employment service staff, it must be asked: what value is this adding and how can we increase this still further?

The assessment phase outlined here clearly has many potential linkages to the audit methodologies discussed specifically in the context of information holdings. However, at this stage what is primarily being considered is the way in which employees work within, and potentially contribute to, the organisation; therefore the benefits are perhaps most clearly allied with concepts of maximising the value and impact of the internal knowledge base. To ask fundamental questions concerning how you use your people remains a widely neglected area of management across all sectors but particularly so in the public sector operating environment. When considering the role of public sector employees, undertaking such a wide-ranging assessment exercise and framing its outcomes and recommendations in respect of a cost/benefit analysis remains a largely alien concept. However, it is clear that, without this vital stage in developing a clear focus on the type of organisation that can best serve emerging models of public service delivery, the potential contribution of the employee-asset base can never be adequately developed.

Design

In the two stages we have considered, aspects of *clarification* have been recommended as being an essential component, inasmuch as they represent a focus upon where the organisation *wants to be*. The *assessment* phase presents the opportunity for analysing where the organisation currently *is*. Taken together, these two elements should provide the genesis of a road map for plotting a way forward in *designing* appropriate methodologies for closing the gap between articulated service aspirations and the reality of current operating mechanisms. At this point, senior-level strategists who understand and are committed to the development of public services which will better utilise their information and knowledge assets will typically face three choices:

- To issue statements and papers which set out their vision of a new organisational culture but without conjoint investment in communicating with and training all levels of staff to take their place within the 'new' organisation. This is typically the public sector approach to implementing change that impacts upon people, and not surprisingly it is a methodology which can bring about only limited returns in respect of service change or improvement. Indeed, there are very real dangers that such an approach may serve to widen the gap between the organisation's aspirations and its actual operating position.
- A second, and again commonly deployed, public sector strategy is to recognise the need for change and, in deciding upon new methodologies and structures, typically to ignore the internal assessment phase of the change process. What will commonly result from this approach are strategies and structures informed very largely by an external focus, typically upon other types of organisations, which show little or no awareness of the actual structures and cultures currently prevalent within the public service organisation under consideration. As a result of this somewhat skewed development process, entirely inappropriate service designs can result, which may in fact serve to reduce rather than enhance opportunities – and willingness – to drive forward the development of an information- and knowledge-'rich' culture.
- The third option available is to ensure that the internal *clarification* and *assessment* phases have been carried out, and to then seek to analyse any gap that may exist between the type of organisation that is aspired to and the way in which people are currently working. There is certainly much to be said, at this point, for seeking to draw in ideas from other types of organisation, or from best practice observed in other countries. However, this should be treated only as *design* input rather than service blueprint, and must be set within the context of understanding the way in which your own employees currently work and what it is that your organisation is aspiring to achieve. This approach is one which supports real *creativity*, but it is a creativity that is firmly rooted in an understanding of the human capital employed within the organisation, and the degree of change that is required of them.

For a *design* phase to be meaningful it must therefore be underpinned by understanding at senior level of exactly what is being undertaken. Only then is it really possible to advocate the creation of programmes and mechanisms which can yield successful information and knowledge outcomes, delivered by all levels of employees. So what does it mean to create an organisation where the open and sharing cultures previously discussed can flourish?

Looking at formal organisational communication flows and structures is a useful way of beginning to understand the way in which barriers to, or support for, information and knowledge sharing already exist. The scenario building approach, discussed in earlier chapters, can be a useful device at this stage for achieving understanding of current practice. So, for example, in a revenue or taxation office scenario, what are the inter-office and intra-departmental communication flows that follow from the first reporting of a client death? Working through such an example, whether the focus is upon the external client or internal processes, is probably the best way of considering what mechanisms currently exist for recording information, the protocols for sharing it with other interested departments, both internally and externally, the duplication that can occur, and the facilities that exist for recording and acting upon issues that arise.

Worked scenarios serve to provide accessible mechanisms for considering how things could be done differently, how better processes and outcomes might be achieved. However, such considerations are not usually something that can be left entirely to a group of senior managers or to external consultants, although the input of both groups may, at various points, be absolutely critical. The design of new ways of working to engender and support the evolution of the type of culture that we have been discussing in this chapter cannot, as we have already stated, simply be 'bolted on'. Nor should any proposed changes be moved to full implementation stage without at least some restricted-scale piloting of new practices. However, even getting to the piloting stage requires considerable attention to be devoted to engaging key organisational employee groups in the ideas generation process. Excluding people assets from the idea-generation and testing processes is, almost at the outset, to negate any aspirations for the achievement of the type of operating culture upon which IKM is dependent. Yet how can you successfully involve your people if they have not been used to a culture that welcomes and encourages participation?

In the first instance, given that public sector organisations are typically large, complex operating structures, it would be advisable for preliminary design-stage work to focus upon one particular location or function in order to assess the type and scale of change required. Having done this, it is most likely that multiple methodologies will be deployed to produce a model for testing. The methodologies used might be those of information and communications flow audits, scenario-building and perhaps, at a slightly later stage, the use of individual and team-based employee inputs to consider current practice in the light of service aspirations. Taking these data, it should then be possible for the IKM project team, if such a group has been established at senior level, to develop a prototype of what new practice might look like.

Implementation

Designing new methods of working which seek to make better use of people resources is not a precise activity, nor is it a naturally rapid one. As we have said, once politicians have identified a particular change priority, public sector organisations are typically not able to devote sufficient time and often requisite resources to engaging in the analysis, design and testing phases required to ensure some likelihood of success. However, when discussing this type of cultural change, it is clear that in the medium and longer term the engendering of the type of organisation that properly utilises its human capital assets is likely to be critically important in developing models of public service which are responsive, and indeed anticipate change, in ways that present structures and cultures neither encourage nor facilitate. Thus, what is needed now is for senior and ambitious public service managers to be anticipating the change agenda of the future and realising that ultimately success may be dependent upon the work that they do *now*, on the development of information- and knowledge-supportive structures.

Implementation of pilot or prototype mechanisms should not be a covert activity; to adopt such an approach is to invite those upon whom you depend for feedback and success to feel threatened or cynical, or perhaps both. If, at the design stage, you have involved key individuals, drawn from all levels of the pilot area, into early discussions of the vision of what you want to achieve and of the limitations or barriers presented by existing structures or systems, then at least you can move forward a proposed new method of working, with a 'mandated in-house' label, either explicitly stated or implied. A pilot phase is reliant, above all else, upon data gathering throughout the designated life cycle of the trial. Some of this may be gathered by covert means, possibly through the use of a 'mystery shopper'-type methodology, particularly in instances where the changes are impacting upon the external client. Fundamentally what this is suggesting is that, parallel to the implementation stage of change, there must be an emphasis upon *monitoring*.

Monitoring

If effective methodologies for better using employees as public service assets are to be developed, there is little to be gained, in respect of achieving longer-term cultural change, from simply deploying pilot studies, whether on a small or larger scale, and simply letting them run. Implementation without ongoing monitoring and appropriate interventions throughout the 'project' life cycle, from first development through to final evaluation, is never going to allow for adequate analysis of impacts upon employees and upon the type and quality of service that result from the changes trailed.

In essence, there is a need to investigate how changed processes impact upon the way in which employees relate to one another and to the organisation as a whole. If the goal of changes being put forward is to achieve a dynamic and continuously evolving culture of information and knowledge exchange and use, then there is a need to assess the extent to which this is actually happening. Thus, monitoring is not exclusively about gathering data to evaluate the achievement or otherwise of task-specific goals, but in this case it must be linked to monitoring performance in relation to the overarching information and knowledge strategy. What you want to know is whether you have been able to design methodologies for working which change the employees' perceptions of themselves, and which encourage and even expect them to communicate and share information and ideas in ways which may be totally alien to previous methods of working.

While you may feel, on reaching the end of these five steps, that much time and not a few resources have been invested in moving forward the issue of human capital-focused cultural change, there is no guarantee that you will automatically have arrived at a model of behaviour or practices which can be rolled out in training and communications programmes throughout the organisation on a once-only basis. Much more likely is an initial outcome that will highlight particular areas or practices as needing addressing at an early stage, thus providing input into the development of organisation-wide training, development and even induction practices. The cultural change envisaged is therefore more likely to evolve over time, supported by informed and supportive senior managers, upon whom the onus for championing and driving forward the realisation of this fundamental change must fall.

Developing information and knowledge 'champions'

Although much of the focus of this chapter has concerned recognising and acting upon the need to ensure that employees, at all levels, understand and are involved in the deployment of IKM strategies, this is not to negate in any way the critical importance of identifying senior-level 'champions' to drive forward this change. The concept of a 'champion' is resonant with much of the Total Quality Management (TQM) literature that emerged in the 1980s. However, in respect of IKM, and in a public sector context especially, the pivotal importance of achieving a senior-level appointment to lead developments in this area is absolutely critical to the achievement of tangible and far-reaching success. TQM theory espoused many views which suggested that 'champions' did not necessarily need to be at the top of the organisation: rather, they were to be selected, or naturally 'emerge', on the basis of a range of factors which focused upon the degree of influence which they were held to have within their immediate workplace community. However, there is little evidence to support the sustained adoption or indeed success of this approach, and its adoption in respect of IKM would be likely to result in confusion and incoherence at the implementation and monitoring stages of the change process.

Issues around leading and driving forward IKM strategies should be considered in respect of current and ongoing debates around the skills and competencies required by *everyone* in a society, defined by the scope and scale of technological and organisational change that is the reality of modern life. In 1998, the Chatham House Forum issued a report taking a UK-centric perspective on possible areas of development until the year 2020; it was predicted that everyone will need to be able to deal with increasing complexity and will require the skills to navigate around less structured organisations and situations: 'Learning methods of handling this complexity will be crucial, and will involve ways of acquiring and using information' (Chatham House Forum 1998: 1). While the issues alluded to here have societal as well as organisational importance, the framework of our focus on the need for IKM leadership – what they serve to do in this context – is to point towards the scale of the undertaking required, for what is actually being proposed is driving forward a new model of employee engagement with the organisation.

As yet, looking across any sector there are few examples of the senior-level appointments that have been referred to here, with the one major exception to this being the practice emerging in management consultancy firms. Here, as we have seen, it has become increasingly normal to see chief knowledge officers (CKOs) operating at the most senior level. As yet, despite some emerging debate in the area, there is little evidence to suggest that public sector appointments have been structured to recruit or develop people into such roles. Analysis of the literature in the IKM area gives few clues as to what is actually required of a senior manager in this area; however, one rare definition is that put forward by Stewart, who suggests that a senior-level information and knowledge manager must be: 'part librarian, part entrepreneur and part cruise-ship social director' (Stewart 1995: 76). More recently, in a research report investigating the skills and competencies required of knowledge managers, Oxbrow and Abell have put forward a more comprehensive, and indeed somewhat daunting, list of key skills and attributes which senior level IKM personnel are felt to require:

Business/management skills

Management of change	Understanding of operating environment
Project management	Facilitation

Marketing   Communication
Leadership   Negotiation
Networking

Team skills

Team leader   Team building
Team player   Interpersonal skills

Human resource skills

Training and development   Human psychology
Motivation   Coaching

KM Skills

Theoretical knowledge   Experience of implementation
KM process development   Understanding of KM-specific ICT
                              applications
Journalism

IM skills

Sourcing and accessing external information
Sourcing and acquiring internal information
Organisation/structuring of information
Database design   Information analysis
Understanding of legal issues such as copyright and data protection

IT skills

Understanding of office systems
Familiarity with external electronic sources
Management of internal databases and intranet applications
Ability to evaluate software applications

Education

First degree   Postgraduate degree, IKM focused if possible
Evidence of ongoing training and development in associated areas

Personal attributes

Strategic thinking

Image:	Professional
	Practical – competence in problem-solving
	Tactical
	Sensitivity and vigilance
Creativity:	Imaginative
	Initiative
	Flexibility
	Lateral thinking
Interpersonal:	Influential
	Diplomatic
	Persuasive
	Engendering trust
	Approachable
	Confident
Involvement:	Interest, curiosity
	Motivation
	High levels of responsibility and willingness to accept accountability

(Oxbrow and Abell 1999: 16)

Taken together, the definitions and descriptions outlined here suggest that, above all, senior-level IKM champions have to be multi-skilled. Adept managers certainly, but also in full command of a complex information and knowledge asset brief, with personal skills and the confidence to persuade and inspire others to adopt strategies that will deliver the dynamic culture required to make managed innovation an ongoing reality. So where in a public sector operating environment does one actually find such people? If we consider emerging practice in other sectors, then the trend is definitely one which sees a majority of such CKO posts being appointed from an internal pool of candidates, although increasingly there is a discernible rise in external recruitment activity.

Appointing a champion of information and knowledge management activity is far from a straightforward exercise. If a branch of public adminis-tration wished to recruit a senior-level accountant or lawyer, for example, there would be a base line of qualifications and experience that could be specified in some detail. However, in seeking to make a CKO appointment, whether drawing upon internal and/or external pools of candidates, what type of background, experience and qualifications can be specified with any degree of accuracy? There is no short, neat answer to this; as yet there are very few academic qualifications that specifically equip students to take up such roles, so requiring the possession of such a 'badge' of competency may be overly limiting. Also, of course, one has to consider the provenance of the person specification emerging: if it has been prepared as a result of less than well-informed political or senior manager level 'recognition' of information and knowledge issues, then there is an inherent danger that the type of person being sought will have a skills base skewed by perception rather than reality. Thus, what might well emerge is the creation of a senior-level information systems post, or a human resource manager with a slightly expanded brief.

When looking at issues that need to be taken on board when moving to create good practice in the area of IKM within public administration structures, a further important consideration is the shelf-life of designated champion posts. If the theory propounded actually holds up in practice, what should happen over time is the elimination of the need for specified posts in the information and knowledge areas. After all, what we have been discussing is fundamentally about reengineering the operational culture of public services; after this has been achieved, there should be little need for formal management structures to remain in place. However, theory and reality do not always follow perfectly symmetrical patterns of behaviour, and just as government departments and agencies retain senior-level managers to oversee and develop functions such as financial management, training and development, client service and administration, so too does it seem likely that, once established, the need for continuous steering of IKM issues will emerge as an ongoing senior-level responsibility.

Given that there appears to be a problem of supply of IKM 'champion' material discernible across all sectors of the economy, it is likely that the public sector, which cannot always compete on salary and bonus packages available in other areas, will have to look internally to develop personnel with the portfolio of skills discussed in this chapter. How they do this depends, of course, on existing approaches to senior staff development within each particular country, authority or agency. Certainly it would seem sensible that all programmes of middle and senior-level management development should include some opportunity for issues of IKM to be raised, so that at least emerging tranches of managers are aware of key issues and of their roles in relation to them. But how can the pivotal figures in moving IKM from rhetoric into practice be recruited and developed by the public sector?

Developing public sector managers at a senior level almost invariably means drawing upon a relatively small pool of available talent. Strategically, when considering personnel planning and issues of leadership of areas of activity it is important to articulate or profile the type of person who is most likely to succeed in a given area. As we have discussed in relation to the skills and attributes of IKM managers, it is the general management, communication, team building and other 'people' skills that are as important as – if not more important than – the overtly IKM specialist skills base identified. Therefore, it may well follow that successful IKM managers can be developed 'in-house' by public sector organisations if consideration is given to the way in which skills-specific development can be incorporated into established training and development programmes.

Globally a number of approaches to senior-level public employee development are evident. In many countries including Canada, the United States, Singapore, France and the United Kingdom, it is common for high-calibre graduates to be recruited into public services and for formal and in some cases 'fast-track' approaches to their development to be adopted. Often, the model for development may be an internally resourced training and education stream such as the UK's Civil Service College and Local Government Training Board. It is also common for partnership arrangements with other training providers, such as universities and consultancies, to be commissioned to deliver 'tailor-made' packages, or to sponsor students to follow taught MBA programmes. However, very few of these approaches have yet been harnessed to ensure that there is an awareness of IKM-specific development issues within a more general focus upon management development. In the short term, it is likely that some personnel may be drafted in from other sectors to provide leadership in this area as demand for senior-level IKM managers grows within the public sector. But perhaps more importantly, public sector managers who recognise the career opportunities will increasingly seek to take advantage of emerging education and training opportunities in this area, in order to leverage their own career opportunities. In this way, the IKM 'champions' needed to drive forward tangible changes in information and knowledge attitudes and behaviours are likely to emerge over time. However, it may be true to say that the greatest career advancement opportunities will be available to those who are able to provide leadership in these areas at an early stage.

Developing the 'front line'

Having argued that the achievement of success in IKM is, in the first instance, largely dependent upon the quality of leadership associated with driving forward related change agendas, it is vital to acknowledge that very little can actually be achieved without the co-operation of all levels of employees. Developing an information- and knowledge-rich public sector operating culture requires that all those involved in managing and delivering services understand and benefit from processes for improving the recognition and management of information and knowledge assets. To achieve such a cultural shift requires something beyond visionary and charismatic leadership, that 'something' being an acknowledgement of the role of people within the organisation and a concomitant commitment to communicating with and providing appropriate training for the various groups within the staffing establishment.

A common approach to ensuring that staff are familiar with changing organisational priorities and aspirations is the use of multi-channel methods of communicating the same message from a senior manager to all members of staff. However, given the size and geographical spread of most public sector organisations, such expressions of intent, vision or refocused mission must be of questionable efficacy in respect of their actual impact upon the culture of service management and delivery. What is much more likely to bring about desired changes is to consider the methods used for facilitating communication to and between groups of staff, and, further, to look at the way in which induction, training, development and performance review systems can be utilised to support the development of an IKM-supporting operating culture.

It is probably true to say that, in a public sector organisation employing five thousand people, only a very small proportion of the total staff need to have any theoretical understanding of what IKM *is*. However, there is a very real requirement to move to a position where all five thousand of these employees follow and benefit from work processes that enable them to operate more efficiently and effectively through better access to and use of information and knowledge, held within or externally accessible to the organisation.

A number of foundation stages may be adopted as the organisation seeks to move to a more IKM-focused mode of operation. A first step is to look at the existing communication channels utilised by staff and to consider the ways in which they are currently used. Typically, what may be found is that, even where relatively sophisticated ICT applications are widely accessible via common operating platforms, no procedures have ever been established to promote or require their use, and this may be an area where some element of 'quick win' can be achieved by looking at ways in which information and knowledge exchange can be easily facilitated. It should also be possible to review recruitment and induction procedures for new employees to ensure that the principles of IKM are introduced at an early stage – again, not in respect of abstract theory, but rather more in terms of introducing good work practices. From a point of considering staff development at its commencement, in terms of induction, much consideration should be given to the design of ongoing staff development programmes, where similar concepts of good work practice, based upon IKM principles, should be engendered, and also held up for some discussion and dialogue.

However, two factors are likely to be critical in ensuring the embedding of IKM within public sector operational contexts. The first is that good practice must be evident among all levels of management; there is little point in requiring that front-line employees adopt a new way of working and embrace a culture that is based upon a preparedness to share and exchange information and ideas, if more senior staff prove reluctant to embrace similar ways of working or demonstrate that their commitment to IKM is only 'solid' as long as what is being shared and exchanged is positive and in alignment with their own particular views.

The second critical success factor is to demonstrate that the adoption of IKM principles is regarded seriously by the organisation. This is done by including some review of IKM attitudes and behaviour within the annual performance review process that is now common for employees in public sector organisations. Undertaking review and monitoring of individual and team performance in respect of IKM is perhaps the best way to demonstrate, and in turn embed, the degree of top-level commitment to developing new ways of working. Engaging with the performance review process represents one of the best opportunities available to the organisation for learning about the way its human resources regard information and knowledge-based processes and structures. Properly constructed review programmes should enable the employee to consider the ways they ensure that IKM practices work for the benefit of the service as a whole, as well as providing valuable opportunities for mapping where blockages and barriers are perceived to occur.

Extracting maximum value from existing procedures such as performance review is undoubtedly an approach to developing IKM within the public sector organisation, and can bring about changes. However, as with all aspects of managing your people within a culture that aspires to utilise information and knowledge assets in new and better ways, little progress can be made if there is only superficial commitment to engaging in an organisational learning and development process. Cynicism and initiative weariness are prevalent in almost every sector but perhaps particularly so in those organisations which operate within the public sector, and such responses to matters of IKM will undoubtedly emerge if there is little evidence from the most senior levels that the changes proposed are actually something that they themselves believe in: this, then, must surely be the key to achieving success in reengineering organisational culture along IKM principles.

Chapter 6

ICTs as tools of IKM

In our discussions of issues around the theories and applications associated with information and knowledge management, the role of information and communications technologies, together with the associated misunderstandings, have been referred to with some regularity. However, despite some of the problems of emphasis that have been identified and discussed, in essence it is possible to argue that issues of IKM and indeed, more fundamentally, of focusing upon the dynamic for change in a public sector context, have been driven forward to a very great extent by the emergence of new 'enabling' technologies. The momentum for organisational change, charted from the emergence of the first widespread adoption of ICTs for information storage and processing in the late 1970s, has resulted in a fundamental reconceptualisation of what it means to be a service-orientated organisation. If we were to look back from a perspective of some three decades hence, it would be possible to chart pressures for change in public sector structures emerging from the wider societal impact of technologies where, for a majority of populations in developed economies, these had served to alter what was understood by *space* and *time*.

What is meant by the allusion to space and time is the way in which the psychology of interface and expectation between the individual and the service organisation has been altered through change mediated by the power of ICTs. So, in a public sector context, it is possible to argue that political enthusiasm for, and public expectations of, services that mirror operations such as telephone- and Internet-based banking, particularly in respect of access, are evidence of societal evolution rather than revolution. Thus, the focus of this chapter is to consider some of the key ICT applications that are increasingly being deployed to facilitate a change in the way in which public sector services operate. Such trends, often referred to under the generic term 'electronic government', are in fact almost always reliant for their success upon some element of properly thought-through information and/or knowledge management theory, although it has only been in the late 1990s that any pattern of evidence linking these concepts with ICT applications can be found in the public sector. At the end of this chapter we will consider the example of Brisbane City Council, which has developed an integrated and technology-enabled approach to delivering citizen-focused services through structuring service delivery modes to make better use of employee resources. This example, which demonstrates what can be achieved through a properly considered deployment of call centre, Intranet and web-based technologies, is responding to the demands of a client base who have become used, through engagement with other areas of life, to doing business remotely and at times convenient to them as the customer rather than within the confines of office hours. Such a model of practice provides, at least in part, a template of how a majority of public services may actually look in the decade to come.

ICTs: a 'tool' of IKM

Within any organisational context the proper place to position the strategic development and deployment of ICTs is to ensure that they are regarded as tools, as *enablers*, rather than *drivers*, of change. Too often, influential commentators have embedded the technology at the heart of the change process, a view at least partly challenged by Hammer, who argues that:

> The watchwords of the decade are innovation and speed, service and quality ... Instead of embedding outdated processes in silicon and software, we should obliterate them and start over. We should reengineer our businesses to use the power of modern information technology to radically redesign our business processes in order to achieve dramatic improvements in their performance.
>
> (Hammer 1990: 104)

So while technological applications are clearly important in organisational structures, whether commercial businesses or public sector services and operations, they should not obliterate from view the clear need to think through *what it is that you want the technology to help you to do*. In IKM-focused operations there is therefore a need to clearly articulate in strategy and planning documents what specific information and knowledge goals and changes can be enabled through the use of technologies. Such an approach, although possibly liable to accusations of being nothing more than much-maligned 'common sense', is not only critical for achieving success in respect of IKM developments but also, vitally, capable of ensuring that investment decisions are properly focused on organisational needs and aspirations, rather than simply reflecting what the technology is deemed to be capable of. Thus, moving towards the adoption of an IKM-centric focus upon public sector management should in practice mean a move to invert the dominant current model of public sector developments, largely driven by capabilities presented by technologies, and arriving instead at a position where technologies are assessed in respect of 'fit' between their potential and what the organisation wants to achieve. Such a perspective, together with the dilemmas represented by the dominance of one mode of operation, is summarised forcefully by Davenport who suggests: 'While millions of high-tech entrepreneurs and bureaucrats work 16-hour days to improve information technology, virtually no one works on information behaviour and effect' (Davenport 1996: 1). Counteracting this imbalance, is, at least in part, one of the challenges for those leading IKM developments in the public sector operating environment.

While this text does not aim to put forward anything approaching a comprehensive review of ICT developments that might conceivably impact upon or support the moving forward of IKM strategies, it is nonetheless important to consider some of the main tools currently available to those developing change agenda in our area of interest. To briefly summarise those which appear, at the outset of the twenty-first century, to be capable of delivering the greatest impact, we should consider the potential of: communications technologies, in particularly the role of telephone-based communications; web-based approaches which include both Internet and Intranet applications; interactive media, including kiosks and digital television; and finally, the use of intelligent agent software. Overarching these applications there must be a further critical element of review and evaluation, not only marrying technologies with what the organisation wants to achieve in respect of IKM, but also achieving a proper degree of focus upon the key issue of *usability* – that is, assessing whether, in practice, IKM strategies, as enabled by ICTs, deliver ways of working within or interacting with the public sector organisation in a manner which represents a qualitative improvement.

The Internet and web-based technologies

It is perhaps somewhat ironic that the now ubiquitous World Wide Web (www), which in the space of less than a decade has contributed to an emerging awareness of the role of information in society and of society as something capable of having a global as well as a national construct, has its roots in military intelligence, an environment where both information and knowledge have for centuries been regarded as the key to gaining and retaining strategic and competitive advantage. With a provenance such as this, firmly embedded in one particular aspect of public sector operation, it might be anticipated that applying such technologies for both information provision and service delivery would figure large in the electronic government operating agenda. Indeed, it is possibly true to say that this is the case: in the United States in particular, there is much evidence of public services having a presence on the www. Here the interface provided to the user can serve as a signpost providing access to information, increasing opportunity to submit completed 'electronic forms' and, in pilot studies at least, the ability to complete transactions by making payments via electronic means.

However, in respect of issues around IKM there are two almost polar positions that can be adopted when regarding the likely impact of web-based technologies on public services. The first position sees the Internet and its allied applications as being profoundly empowering, making available information that had previously been accessible only via visits to offices or libraries. However, running counter to this is the notion of the information overload contributing to something that becomes no more than an information 'sewer' – where, paradoxically, the very quantity available, the formats used, the lack of focus on the quality of content, all potentially contribute to a generation of public sector users who are overwhelmed rather than empowered.

The principles explored in the opening chapters of this book, which considered the concepts of defining information and knowledge as assets and developing strategies to promote their successful use and development, have rarely been more notable by their absence than in relation to the public sector stampede towards establishing a presence on the web. However, one well-thought-out example can be seen in Illinois in the United States, where the Gateway project, an Internet-based service, acts to provide a link to the governor's office and related departments. By accessing a web page, citizens are able to: complete vehicle licensing procedures; order official publications and forms; obtain information on land sale and registration; and link to the home pages of other state and national government agencies. While anyone with a personal computer linked to the Internet can access the Illinois Gateway, issues of exclusion have, to some extent at least, been addressed through the installation of a significant number of free public access kiosks throughout the state, where the same level of active engagement can be achieved. Such examples should leave us in no doubt that properly thought-through, web-based technologies offer tremendous opportunities for realising the full potential of IKM-focused strategies in a public sector operating environment.

Telephone-based services: the emergence of the call centre

Possibly the ICT application which has had greatest impact upon service-based industries during the 1990s, and one which is beginning to result in considerable public sector interest and take-up, is the development of call centre based interfaces with external clients. Despite the undoubted growth in public interest in, and access to, computer-driven sources of information and communication, it remains an undisputed fact that it is the telephone which today has by far the greatest levels of public familiarity and access. Drawing together these critical elements of non-threatening public perceptions and widespread technology penetration, the call centre proposition has flourished. It has become increasingly complex in the way in which it can engage in service provision in the commercial sectors, and is now beginning to have significant impact upon the rethinking of aspects of public service structure and delivery modes. However, it is possibly true to say that key drivers for moving towards adoption of this approach have rarely articulated the IKM principles for doing so, instead being couched in terms of leveraging overall efficiency alongside the achievement of cost savings.

However, in briefly considering the example of the financial services sector, we can begin to make sense of the potential contribution of the adoption of such approaches in a public sector context. Apart from the fact that the numbers of customers opting to conduct transactions over the telephone indicates that there is demand for and appreciation of the flexibility that such services offer, it can be argued that there are significant IKM-based reasons for adopting such modes of delivery. In the first instance, it is important to differentiate between types of call centre. To date, many of those emerging in the public sector simply act as information gateways – typically, there may be one national telephone number for social security enquiries, but the service is actually a brokering one, either passing out further telephone contact numbers or generating a request for information to be posted on to the enquirer. Although this is a relatively unsophisticated construct, one should not underestimate the efficiency gains to be made from moving towards the adoption of such practices. By using free-phone or low-charge telephone numbers, the service is not limiting citizen access in any way, yet it is likely to gain considerable efficiency savings by moving much of its first-level information-provision role into a centralised and structured environment.

Such 'simple' call centre approaches certainly make a contribution to the way in which information flows through and from public service structures. However, major opportunities for service development can be missed if a focus upon service and efficiency improvements is not accompanied by an awareness of how the larger organisation can benefit from the information and knowledge flowing into the call centre. Using software packages available, it is relatively straightforward, in this call centre context, to provide a profile of service use, allowing analysis of usage patterns, in terms of the types of query being raised, the timings and the physical locations or origin of the queries. When fed into decision-making processes at a strategic level, such information can serve to ensure that there is at least some awareness of which areas are generating the greatest numbers of queries across a function or service.

Such an approach enables far better IKM outcomes, for base data at least, which can then be further interpreted. Here is a mechanism that can operate across nations or regions within them, and can bypass the barriers of poor recording or sharing mechanisms which exist when such operations are handled largely through local offices. What is therefore represented here, in this very straightforward application of call centre methodologies, is a technology-enabled way of ensuring that core service information is available on a regular basis for the development of awareness and knowledge, at a senior level, of what clients are actually asking for. Developing the sophistication of analysis still further, it is also possible, at an early stage, to map the linkages articulated in their requests between their perceived information needs and the mismatch that may occur within the way that public services are structured.

Importantly, even the most apparently straightforward information-providing call centre application represents considerable opportunities for breaking down some of the traditional barriers that have existed, institutionally at least, between functions internal to one designated department or service and those across the public sector as a whole. However, what must be acknowledged is that, as yet, there are very few examples of public services being able to move fully to address a number of key citizen issues:

> 'Why do I have to call so many places? Why do I have to wait so long? Why can't they solve my problems right here, right now?' These are questions that governments must take seriously. Government must reinvent itself, as other institutions have had to to survive.
>
> (Horton 1994: 6)

The critical reason, of course, why so many locations have to be called and so many delays occur, is that information-sharing mechanisms do not exist to make 'one-stop' service delivery or even information provision a reality in all but a small number of (largely restricted size) examples; and this is setting aside issues around the problematic nature of breaking down barriers that have grown up around public services as largely autonomous operating units within a whole.

The role of more complex call centre approaches in reinventing the way that the public sector is structured to do business is only beginning to emerge. However, if we consider the way in which Singapore – admittedly a relatively small and highly centralised nation-state – has addressed the issues of harnessing certain technologies to move forward public service provision, we can see that call centre applications are at the heart of their vision of developing an integrated mode of transacting government/citizen exchanges:

> Call centres can be used to allow people to call government agencies to obtain information on policies, procedures, services and the status of their applications for permits and licences ... The call centre comprises both interactive voice response systems and customer service officers. Services which are transactional in nature will be provided by interactive systems, while information services will be provided by officers. ... For

information services, it is not necessary to verify the identity of the caller. In fact callers may even wish to remain anonymous. ... One major component of the Government Call Centre project is to put in place the necessary hardware, software and networking infrastructure to support the various call centres ... The customer service officer is able to access back-office host computer systems and databases.

(Burkitt-Gray 1996: 15)

We are left in no doubt that what is critical to the achievement of success in this context is the ability to access information held by a number of discrete service areas. To what extent this is a realistic aspiration for public sector structures in nations which have far larger total populations than Singapore, simply because of the scale of the undertaking represented in making meaningful information interchange a reality, is undoubtedly a critical issue when considering just how far call centres can be utilised within present public sector structures and cost constraints.

If we were in the position today of developing a blueprint for the way in which public services were designed, it is unlikely that the ideal emerging would resemble, to any great extent, the pattern of provision and structures that we see employed to support them now. The structures that we observe today, with tiers of government and stovepipe function-driven patterns of organisation, are a legacy of decades and in some cases centuries of bureaucratic predominance: a dominance which has prevailed in approaches to the adoption of ICTs. Thus, while what we might articulate in our blueprint for better government would be a boundary-free, barrier-reduced, information-sharing type of service, personified by the use of call centre applications capable of making linkages across functional boundaries in order to deliver to the citizen the total service that they would wish to receive, the reality in terms of what can be achieved is hindered by the legacy of the past. Cross-boundary services as opposed to simply information-providing call centres are reliant for their success, as with the Singaporean example, upon being able to link easily into the information holding and handling systems of a number of departments. This is not, in theory at least, an intrinsically problematic position to achieve: for example, if we consider the financial services paradigm, we can see that it is possible in single transactions to achieve interaction between apparently diverse products – your call centre operator may be able to provide status information on your mortgage, pay a bill for you and give a quote on an insurance package, all within the framework of one telephone call. Of course, the reason for this is that such systems have had the benefit of growing from an essentially 'green field' base, where specifications of what the business wanted to do and the technology required were newly commissioned.

The public sector rarely presents us with a technology green field, especially when our goal, as discussed here, is to make possible seamless interactions between different functional or departmental boundaries. To aspire, for example, in a United Kingdom – or one day, perhaps, European Union – context, to deliver boundary-free public services to citizens, whereby they might in the same call make a pensions query, pay an instalment of a tax bill and request information on schools in a certain area, remains a somewhat distant proposition. Distant, not because call centre technologies *per se* are insufficiently developed or robust to underpin such a wide-ranging undertaking, but rather because simply mapping ICT practices across departments and functions is likely to present a picture of chaos and muddle, where incompatibility of various technologies presents the most significant barrier of all to sharing the critical information holdings necessary to make new 'joined-up' modes of public service provision a reality.

In seeking to utilise some of the best technology-enabled reengineering of modes of service delivery, a critical problem for the public sector is the legacy built over the last twenty or more years of largely ignoring the need for common operating platforms across government. Diversity of product choice and of approaches used has resulted in a position where, almost paradoxically, the very technology that has been held up as the driver of more efficient public services is itself a major barrier to achieving the large-scale collapsing of traditional operational boundaries enabled by easy information exchange. Such a position has arisen mainly because little attention has historically been paid to ensuring that ICT purchasing decisions within public services should be made, at least partly, upon the basis of ensuring compatibility with other systems running in related areas of government.

Truly innovative and barrier-reducing call centre applications, operating on a wide scale and serving large populations, remain limited in the extent to which they can be realised; although the necessary information exists in electronic format, the variety of technological applications in existence serves in many cases to prevent the interchange and interaction required to enable a more complex call centre application to work in practice. However, this is not to say that, over time, this position cannot be rectified. Increasingly, we see governments and transnational alliances such as the European Union setting out protocols for ICT compatibility which both give guidance to their own managers, as clients, and – perhaps just as importantly – send out important messages to suppliers regarding what is now expected of them when selling into a public sector context. Over time, and certainly within the next decade, as technologies are superseded it is likely that an operating environment which supports rather than impedes information-sharing will emerge in the public sector environment, and as it does, call centre applications will be at the forefront of delivering far more holistic and citizen-focused modes of operation.

An interesting example of the way in which first steps are being taken by a major United Kingdom government agency, at least in respect of testing out how the call centre model of operation might impact upon major service realignment, is that of the Inland Revenue's first call centre, based in East Kilbride in Scotland. However, some of the issues alluded to previously become all too apparent when reviewed in an applied context, as Burkitt-Gray observes:

> Ministers have said again and again that they aspire to ensuring that public services are comparable with the best that the commercial sector has to offer. East Kilbride is the Inland Revenue's first attempt at exploring the implications behind those promises ... Nationally the Revenue is not committing itself to adopt call centres. Indeed, for historical reasons East Kilbride has clear advantages which make it a sensible place for a trial – but perhaps not such a good place from which the rest of the Revenue can learn. For a start, information about most taxpayers who work for Scottish employers is already centralised in East Kilbride. It is called Centre 1, and it has the records of 2.5m taxpayers.
> (Burkitt-Gray 1999: 20)

The scale of this pilot project is perhaps the most significant thing to note about it; handling a full range of employee and employer taxation information for such a large number of individuals represents a considerable undertaking. Yet one lesson is clear from this: the East Kilbride pre call centre operating environment was part of the patchwork of different approaches to Inland Revenue organisation that had grown up across the UK over previous decades, most of which had resulted in a dispersed and more locally based network of offices as the repositories of information on far smaller numbers of clients. To extend this, given positive citizen and employer feedback, would be by no means straightforward, given that the aim would be to merge all information holdings and make them accessible via a range of call centres, operating nationally but not necessarily with any specific geographic links to the client community, as in the East Kilbride exemplar site.

Having overcome the current technology barriers to information sharing, there are likely to be other major cultural and organisational barriers to moving towards the successful adoption of a commercial sector paradigm of integrated call centre use in the public sector operating environment. As Burkitt-Gray observes in his study of the East Kilbride prototype, although managers may boast:

> At the end of a call, our staff always say, 'Is there anything else I can do while we are on the phone?' ... What happens when a caller says: 'I've let you know I've been made redundant. Do I need to tell the Employment Service separately?' Or: 'I've said I'm taking maternity

leave. Can you pass it on to the Benefits Agency so I'll get child benefit?'
That would be joined-up government.

(Burkitt-Gray 1999: 21)

Call centres may certainly have a role to play in delivering this vision of a
new and joined-up mode of service provision, but what must be clearly
understood is the imperative for all such ICT deployment to be underpinned
by a sound framework for understanding and utilising the information and
knowledge assets which comprise their resource base and fundamentally
their *raison d'être*.

The role of the Intranet in IKM

In their 1998 discussion of how the importance of Intranet technologies can
be defined and contextualised, White *et al.* report: 'Within this changing
economic environment, and in an increasingly fast and competitive global
market, the concepts of knowledge management and of Intranet technology,
have come to dominate headlines in the business press over the past year or
so' (White *et al.* 1998:3). Evolving from operating protocols first used in
Internet applications, an Intranet is now commonly referred to as the
internal information and knowledge engine of all types of organisations,
networked across offices, locations and, in some instances, national boundaries. Properly constructed, it should offer, at appropriate levels of security
clearance, a way of empowering an employee to navigate the most suitable,
and value-adding path through the organisation's operating structures, information holdings and knowledge base. It is a tool of such potential
importance that in a 1998 research report, KPMG argued that:
'Organisations which (by the year 2000) do not have an Intranet are likely to
be at a competitive disadvantage' (KPMG 1998a: 3). Such exhortations have
not been lost on politicians: certainly, at the close of the twentieth century
there was a marked increase in activity to ensure that public sector organisations responded to the challenges of using technology in such a way that
clear synergies between IKM and technologies could be seen to be operating. This suggested, perhaps for the first time, the role of an ICT
application in maximising the value of internally held information and
knowledge which should be accessible across the organisation. However, as
yet there are few examples of truly integrative and sophisticated Intranet
deployment in global public services, but this is not to say that, as the
methodology of deployment matures, the current relatively unsophisticated
applications observable in the public sector cannot develop into potentially
powerful IKM tools, as we shall discuss in relation to a module of Intranet
evolution.

Within this evolutionary context, it is possibly true to say that the term
'Intranet' is used rather more generically than most observers on the subject

admit. Indeed, it is helpful in a public sector analysis and planning context to consider the five-stage approach to development posited by White *et al.*, who chart the main stages of development observed in applied contexts where there would appear to be rich learning opportunities for those organisations considering embarking upon such projects:

Stage 1: Internal publishing

The majority of Intranets start as a mechanism for the internal distribution of documents, such as manuals, procedures, staff lists, etc. Often the documents are loaded onto the Intranet without any change to the format or structure used for the paper version, with the result that they are actually quite difficult to access and use.

The initiative for launching the Intranet usually originates in the IT department, sometimes with the encouragement of the human resources department. Drivers are not business strategies, knowledge management strategies or information strategies, and the content is rarely designed to meet user needs or to support business processes. Even with good internal marketing, the usage is low, the costs can be high and the return on investment difficult to see or prove.

The justification for implementing these Intranets are usually the cost-savings of not having to print and circulate the documents, and the ease of updating. This may be valid justification but if the documents are not well used in print format (as is often the case with this sort of material) then it is highly unlikely that they are going to be used any more frequently in electronic format.

The end of this stage is usually a feeling of disappointment on the part of all concerned that the vision, often hyped-up, has not been achieved. In fact it was just a vision, and there was no formal set of objectives developed against which resources could be allocated and progress measured (White *et al.* 1998: 10).

This early stage of adoption displays many of the characteristics of poor co-ordination and lack of strategic thinking and planning that have been previously discussed in this text. The adoption of applications such as Intranets, which result in nil or extremely limited benefits for their public sector user, is most likely to result from ill-focused and poorly understood information- and knowledge-driven specifications. To install the technology is never going to be enough: to utilise it successfully through gaining widespread adoption of working practices based upon access to the applications must be the goal, but if there is no progress from the position articulated at Stage 1 there can be little real justification, in IKM terms at least, for the adoption of such an approach.

Stage 2: Redefining the objectives

What soon starts to emerge is that different business units may have different 'views' of the content to reflect their particular needs and uses. Even more obvious are the resources required to update the content, and to convert information that has not previously existed in an electronic format. It is at this stage that a degree of realism, and even disappointment, starts to creep into the discussions, as it becomes clear that the Intranet is more than another IT project, and needs to support staff in achieving business objectives.

The result is often that responsibility for the content and management of the Intranet moves to individual departments ... Another feature of this stage is that attention starts to be paid to integration of internal and external database information ... Usually internal databases of client or product information are given early priority.

Stage 2 is still very much an information publishing model, the difference from Stage 1 is that the content is increasingly driven by the needs of the business, rather than the provision of electronic versions of corporate level material, and that there is a higher degree of departmental involvement in content creation (White *et al.* 1998: 11).

Although some of the language used is suggestive of a commercial business environment, the underlying rationale for considering ways in which Intranet usage can become far more firmly embedded within operating cultures remains highly relevant to a public sector operating context. Where examples of Intranet development currently exist in this sector, it is certainly possible to plot their approaches as being typically in transition from Stage 1 to Stage 2. If we consider the largest UK public sector Intranet project, launched in 1998 under the auspices of the Cabinet Office in partnership with a commercial network provider, the Government Secure Intranet (GSI), although still in its early stages, shows some evidence of maturing into at least a Stage 2 application. Offering a secure operating environment, the ultimate intention is to support collaborative working through information access and exchange across departmental boundaries. However, at launch and in the following eighteen months, the GSI exhibited important evidence of 'bedding in' and the establishment of a culture where electronic media became increasingly accepted modes of accessing information and knowledge assets, admittedly at an internal operating level. The likelihood is that, as this increasingly Intranet-familiar and -comfortable operating culture emerges, subsequent stages of development will be less problematic to achieve.

Stage 3: Collaborative working

Stage 3 marks quite a major shift in focus, as now the Intranet starts to be used to exchange knowledge, largely about and between people. This is also the stage at which content starts to be created specifically for the Intranet, such as descriptions of projects, expertise databases, and consistently formatted cv's. This exchange of knowledge has always been the primary objective of the Intranets developed by the major management consultancies, where the most valuable information is the expertise of the consultants and details of the projects that they have worked on. This stage marks a very important shift in the culture of the organisation, as the process of exchanging knowledge can be very threatening if not handled correctly. One result is that human resources departments start to become increasingly interested in the benefits of Intranets.

Also at this stage companies often start to integrate groupware applications into the Intranet, such as meeting scheduling, discussion groups and eventually document preparation. More attention is paid to providing considered access to external sources of information (White *et al.* 1998: 12).

Thus Stage 3 can definitely be seen as a maturing period for Intranet applications. However, what is apparent is, of course, that to move to this position and beyond requires that there is a real and driving vision at senior level, underpinning what is wanted by the organisation. What this relates to at a fundamental level is the need to have a clearly articulated IKM strategy that is both managed and communicated across and between the various public sector levels and strands of operation. Without this, the collaboration or 'joining up' that the rhetoric and literature of public sector organisational reform has adopted as its governing mantra cannot be expected to be achieved.

Stage 4: Business process integration

By Stage 4 the Intranet has become sufficiently ubiquitous and useful that it almost ceases to have a specific identity at all. Users begin to identify the services and resources that they have access to, rather than the technical infrastructure which supports them.

Stage 5: From Intranet to extranet

An extranet gives yet another dimension to the Intranet, enabling information distribution, collaboration and transactions to take place with external partners. For extranets to be effective, legal and safe there are many new issues that need to be addressed, such as technical issues relating to standards, firewalls, and security and business strategies relating to the level of collaboration with both suppliers and customers (White *et al.* 1998: 12).

In these final two stages we see the cultural embedding of the Intranet as an internal driver of IKM practice and, importantly, consideration being given to the ways in which such applications can be utilised in relationships with other organisations. The development of extranets is likely to become more and more important in a public sector context, where increasingly there is a globally observable trend towards the contracting of certain functions to external parties, partnerships with both the private and voluntary sectors, and agency relationships between different tiers of government itself, as well as more generally understood procurement activities

However, a major caution in relation to this, and to Intranet developments more generally, is that they must be properly thought through, not simply the result of some identified imperative to replicate commercial sector practice. Communication and education processes are fundamental to the success of Intranets and associated applications. Further, in order to be successful, they must have been framed in respect of a clearly articulated vision of what is actually being aspired to, and need to demonstrate from the outset that their adoption is driven by understanding of how the organisation is structured and the ways in which co-operation and collaboration can be enabled. Without such an operating 'map', Intranet technologies are likely to realise only a very small part of their potential.

Kiosk-based services: dinosaurs or demiurge?

As with call centre applications, kiosk-based delivery of information and services has received much attention in the debate around likely vehicles for delivering 'electronic government'. Perhaps the main argument in favour of the adoption of kiosks is the opportunities that are afforded for locating them in 'non-traditional' service areas, such as shopping malls, pedestrianised precincts and public libraries, where an emphasis upon raising levels of citizen awareness and access to kiosk-based services can be explored outside the normal remit of government, agency or council offices. Kiosks are thus often viewed as tools in the democratisation of citizen access to both information and service provision within the public sector.

There are reasonable questions which should be asked around the extent to which the notion of the kiosk has been superseded, in purely technological terms, by the emergence of Internet-based access to information, increasingly available to citizens in their own homes, and the emerging digital television applications that may, in the relatively short term, serve to personalise still further public access to all tiers of government services. However, what is most important about the concept of the kiosk, and which may well serve to extend the life of such propositions in service terms, is their very visibility. Kiosk applications such as those now particularly common in Spain and Singapore, located in residential areas, in places where people socialise, around schools and retail outlets, do potentially serve to send out a message that public services are increasingly citizen-centric. We should not underestimate the issue of location of kiosks and the associated benefits that can accrue from being seen to embed the business of interaction with public services within operating environments which people routinely use.

When considering what kiosks are capable of, we find a tremendous diversity of practice. In North America there have been pockets of considerable investment in using kiosks in service delivery transactions as well as information-providing roles. As Thornton argues:

> International examples abound of effective use of kiosk technology to deliver government services. Perhaps one of the most effective, long-standing implementations is that found in Ontario. Since 1993, a network of self-service kiosks installed throughout the Canadian province has enabled residents to obtain key motor vehicle information and services at more convenient times and locations.
>
> The program, named ServiceOntario, began as a pilot and expanded rapidly. Today, over 60 self-service kiosks allow citizens to:
>
> Renew vehicle registrations
> Pay court and parking fines
> Order custom license plates
> Search driver and vehicle records
> Update change-of-address information
>
> Response to the program has received overwhelming support from citizens, with 94 per cent of users rating the service 'easy to use and enjoyable' ... the ServiceOntario system delivers financial benefits to both parties. As a transaction-based system, the costs of operating come down as the volumes rise and the system becomes increasingly more cost-effective as other government agencies add services. And because the kiosk handles routine, time-consuming procedures, the skills and time of motor-vehicle agency employees can be directed to more important higher-value tasks.
>
> (Thornton 1997: 20)

Important IKM points are raised here primarily because, of course, IKM-based public sector functions do have as their goal the achievement of far more focused, efficient and ultimately effective ways of working. Within this context, then, and considering well-developed examples such as ServiceOntario or the employment services model utilised increasingly by the Australian Centrelink, one can readily build an organisational case for developing and investing in kiosk-based applications. Such approaches have, in practice, demonstrated that they can deliver citizen information, certain types of primarily routine transactions, from employment services through to social security claims, local taxation and even, in the case of the QuickCourt system in Arizona in the USA, information and assistance with the preparation of documentation in small claims and divorce matters.

Increasingly, too, the touch-screen technology provided by kiosks is being complimented by other kiosk 'add-ons': the provision of telephone links may allow contact with the public service department or agency concerned, or, in the case of employment services, vacancy information displayed on screen may then offer the user the opportunity to telephone the prospective employing organisation direct, in order to request additional information or to express interest. The development of robust and more cost-effective video links between kiosks and office locations is also offering an opportunity for expanding and developing the service, mediation and advice-provision aspects of public services through technology-enabled remote access.

However, there are two key concerns around the continuing development of kiosk-based services, responses to which are likely to be influential in deciding whether, in the medium-term, such applications are to be viewed as dinosaurs, supplanted by other more 'focused' uses of technology, or demi-urges at the forefront of IKM-enabled public services. Let us consider the first scenario, which sees kiosks as being simply a stepping-stone on the way to the achievement of public services which are, in effect, delivered to the citizen in their own homes or offices – the ultimate in personal service. The achievement of such a position is, even in the most optimistic calculations, still some years away, and even the most optimistic of champions would have to acknowledge that universal access to ICT tools and full confidence and competence in the skills to use them lie even further in the future.

As a tool for moving public services out from their traditional office bases and harnessing touch-screen option-driven modes of technology provision, the kiosk would appear to have much to offer. However, while there are successful and sophisticated examples of deployment, such as those outlined above, the overall perception of the role and potential of kiosk-based service delivery has been marred by far too many ill-thought-out, costly and ulti-mately pointless examples of deployment. For example, Pollett discusses an interactive kiosk in a United Kingdom local government context, where, using a public library location as a base for what is referred to as a 'One Stop Shop', citizens can check their eligibility for both local and national welfare benefits – at the very least a worthy pilot study, one might think. However, the reality as described by Pollett is somewhat different:

When I visited it, the screen was frozen. I asked Clare, the intelligent and pleasant assistant on the first Stop desk, how to get the kiosk going. Conspiratorially, she said 'Just go round the back and switch off the plug and switch it on again.' She might as well have said: 'Give it a kick.' … The touch-screen kiosk had been in position for just three weeks but, as Clare and her colleagues confirmed, it has already been well used. Particularly by 'kids' who discovered that at certain times it could be used – not that this is the intention – to surf the Internet.

Interestingly the Stop Shop staff had wanted a software program put on their PCs so that they could do face-to-face interviews with clients who needed benefit advice. Instead the Social Justice Unit from the council summarily dumped the kiosk in the shop. Not that the staff are resentful about this. They clearly see that the kiosk is, and will be, of benefit to those who would rather share their personal details with a PC than with another human being using a PC. That's only human, I guess.

But you will need to be an odd type of humanoid to make sense of the software application on this kiosk. It would be helpful if you were a lawyer – considering the complexity of the questions asked by the software on Bamm – Benefits Advice in Multimedia. Try this for instance: 'Does your disability mean that if you worked you would only expect to do or earn 75 per cent as much as a fit person?' … This is the sort of question dreamed up by public sector actuaries and it certainly doesn't make for a very user-friendly front-end, even for an English speaker. For a borough with a large population for whom English is not a first language, it is a definite oversight that Bamm operates only in English.

Quite apart from the complexity of the questions, the text on the screen is hard to read. It is white, against a powder-blue background. Pretty but useless. … also, it told me after I'd completed the quick questionnaire that if I wanted to 'go further', I could 'get advice from the Citizens Advice Bureau, or other agency' – but it didn't tell me where they were.

After you've completed the questionnaire, Bamm plays happy music if you are entitled to benefit and sad music if you're not, treating the process of applying for benefit – often a life and death issue – with a game show mentality.

(Pollett 1999: 28–9)

The message here, of course, is that if kiosks are to be used successfully as a tool of reengineering the way in which the public sector is structured to 'do business', then it has got to be properly thought through. In practice, decisions around using kiosks, call centres, Internet services and Intranets require that fundamental questions must be asked about what it is that you want them to achieve and how they, as tools, contribute to IKM goals organisation-wide and in respect of enhanced citizen interface with public services. Kiosks should not be dismissed out of hand, for in themselves they can be many things: increasingly, technology is offering the possibility not only of making them interactive in a formulaic manner but also, through the convergence of ICT applications, of opening up the possibility for 'real-time' engagement with government officers operating at remote locations.

Such applications are not, of course, without costs, and these can be very significant in terms of both start-up and ongoing maintenance. This is where a further important issue needs to be input into kiosk programme planning and management processes: that of who 'owns' the kiosks and their content. The answer might, initially at least, appear straightforward – if they are public sector kiosks then they are 'owned' by their commissioning agency or department – but what happens to a well-developed kiosk network in the case of Australia, when employment services were to a large extent privatised on a regional basis? Fundamentally, what we see here is the tension between commercial drivers and the tradition of the public sector 'good'. In the case of the Australian Automated Job Search (AJS), a nation-wide network of kiosks was located in shopping malls and libraries as well as employment offices; the underpinning national information-sharing base, whereby vacancy information was made available to all and upon which the kiosk model had been built, was obliterated by the move to a commercial model of operation. Although regional providers were offered the chance to buy into the AJS network, the reality for most was that they chose not to, citing what was perceived as the prohibitive cost of subscribing to the kiosk network, and, less explicitly but perhaps more importantly, a reluctance to share their own employment vacancy information with other providers. Thus, as new models of public/private partnership in service delivery begin to emerge, the role of the kiosk, as potentially the most visible of ICT applications, needs to be carefully thought through regarding content ownership and management: without this, the 'dinosaur' scenario is never far away.

Focusing on usability

Underpinning all IKM theory is the need to articulate what it is that you are seeking to identify and manage, and to move forward only on the basis of having done this and of having made an ongoing commitment to continuous review and evaluation of practice and achievements. When considering the role of ICTs in respect of this continuing process, the danger is that it is the technology which dominates the agenda, rather than considerations of what it might be used to achieve. However, even in instances where IKM has been the primary driver of change, with the technology firmly placed in an enabling role, there has been a substantial history of failure to achieve significant improvements in operations and services. A key reason for this, which may certainly be said to be evident in the discussion of kiosk-based applications, is the apparent failure to focus adequately on issues around what is often termed 'usability'. To adopt a commercial sector example, one would have to acknowledge that it would be very unlikely that a new chocolate bar could reach the market without extensive market research and testing first taking place, to ensure that the proposed new product was likely to meet with approval from potential customers. However, analysis of public sector change agenda, whether impacting internally, externally or through a combination of both, shows an arena in which inadequate focus on the issue of the perceptions of and impact upon users feeds into indifferent and occasionally failing performance; this in turn leads to employee and citizen cynicism – potentially the greatest source of resistance to change itself.

The concept of usability testing or measurement in a public sector ICT context is as yet poorly developed:

> There is too little evidence, however, that practice adopted in the commercial sector – whereby a critical part of the development of products/services, particularly those that involve the deployment of technologies, involves extensive attitude/opinion testing – has been carried over with any real commitment or efficacy into the public sphere. Indeed ... research revealed that constraints of resources and time meant that, in almost all cases of electronic government initiative considered, inadequate pre-testing took place prior to full-scale launch. This was found to be particularly true when considering the deployment of kiosk technologies, where both the end-user interface and the actual location of the interface, key critical success factors, were inadequately trialled prior to deployment. ...
>
> In this context, the concept of ensuring access to, and time for utilising 'usability laboratories', where ergonomic, content and interface aspects of ICTs are tested on potential end-users in carefully monitored situations, is something that should be actively pursued in the public sector. In one instance, a very rare example it must be said, the establishment of such a laboratory by a department in Australia, at cost of some $AU300,000, saved in its first week of operation, projected costs of some $AU500,000. This was achieved by identifying, through work with end-users and front-line employees, that the software under test required modifications in order to improve both its operational efficiency and end-user satisfaction with the interface provided.
>
> (Milner 1999: 70–71)

Taking the time and investing resources to ensure the potential usability and ultimate efficacy of an ICT application, or indeed any significant change of procedure which has an information or knowledge component, does not appear to be a radical proposition. Yet, the evidence suggests that this is a major area of neglect, and a costly one at that: costly in terms particularly of failure or inefficiency being the end-product of implemented change.

Critically, in respect particularly of KM processes, the usability testing and proving stages offer a structured opportunity to engage in proper utilisation of employees as assets, at appropriate phases in their involvement in the process being considered, and also for engaging in dialogue with ultimate end-users, be they individual citizens, other organisations, other government departments or agencies. Rather than being perceived as a cost, IKM managers should be promoting a position that views usability as a key stage in the achievement of ongoing improvement.

Drawing ICTs together – the example of Brisbane City Council (BCC)

Located at the southern tip of Queensland in Australia, Brisbane is a city of some one and a half million residents. In locating itself both nationally and internationally, it sees itself as a trading hub for the Asia–Pacific region. Measured against some key organisational indicators, BCC is the third largest city authority in the world, both in respect of the geographic area that it covers and the complexity of services for which it is responsible – including water, roads and transport. Politicians are elected on a three-yearly basis and are salaried, and there is a directly elected mayor who presides over a 'civic cabinet'. A brief profile such as this is helpful in setting out why there are valuable lessons to be learned from the practice adopted within BCC with regard to IM and, through it, to the rolling out of innovative and successful ways of utilising ICTs to drive forward improvements in service design and delivery.

Taking an historical perspective, it is possibly true to say that up until 1995 BCC had no clear direction on reengineering service provision and was spending in excess of $AU50 million per annum on ICT applications, with no underpinning co-ordination and therefore with much duplication and failure the typical end results of investment. However, with the appointment of a Chief Executive Officer, Robert Carter, leadership and vision around the type of public sector authority that BCC could legitimately aspire to be became almost immediately apparent. One of his first acts was to establish an Information Resource Management Committee under the leadership of another key strategic appointment, Helen Ringrose, which had a mandate to *slow* everything down, initially at least – to take the time to develop an information strategy for the authority and, in support of that, an ICT architecture that would provide a blueprint for all planned changes. Articulation of what the information strategy and the associated architecture were intended to achieve was straightforward: all proposed changes had to meet two key criteria. They must:

- advantage the customer;
- demonstrate the achievement of value for money.

On the basis of this clear vision of how BCC planned to utilise and manage its information assets, a number of key priorities were identified where it was felt that technology could provide a key enabling role. These were:

*   dissemination of internal and external information via the Internet and Intranet;
*   bringing functionality closer to the user;
*   creating environments that are flexible and supportive of change;
*   improved delivery mechanisms (including mobile and remote access).

The setting of such goals was rationalised in both 'political' and organisational terms through focusing upon the expected benefits and outcomes of moving to such an approach. These were couched in terms of leveraging the quality of customer service; bringing about much-needed consistency in respect of both internal and external information delivery; making possible both local and remote information access to citizens; and contributing to an enhanced sense of community within the BCC operating region.

Perhaps the most significant first step on the road to realising a public sector mode of working that prioritised excellence in IM was the creation in 1996 of the BCC call centre. Once this was established across the authority, there were over three hundred telephone contact points that the public might reasonably make use of; between them, they received approximately seven thousand calls per day during tightly defined operating hours. It was decided that consideration of customer contact via the telephone would represent an important first review step in building an effective information architecture. Eschewing an external consultant-intensive approach, BCC staff used a mapping process to understand the scope of the majority of their client calls and developed a Windows-based call management system; by 1997 this had reduced the number of BCC telephone numbers available to the public to some fifteen, with a goal – achieved for the majority of users – of reducing to one single access number by 1999. Again, in 1997 the decision was made to move to a seven-day a week, twenty-four-hours a day operating policy for the call centre. Evaluation of progress made and citizen perceptions of the service delivered revealed that 90 per cent of calls were capable of being handled directly by the call centre 'consultant'; the remaining number of cases could either be linked directly to an appropriate internal contact, or be referred via email to the department or individual required. Additionally, high levels of end-user satisfaction with the system were recorded, which appeared to impact positively on the more general public perception of BCC.

What was most significant about the roll out and success of the call centre approach was the transforming effect that it had upon the organisational culture, and indeed upon external opinions and expectations of BCC services. In organisational architecture terms, the call centre provided the foundations of information-driven change which have allowed the building of other ICT-assisted initiatives. Most importantly, BCC has emerged as a major public sector authority which has a vision of service provision as something that should be accessible at any time and through a diversity of locations. The call centre approach demonstrated that this was a mode of interface to which citizens responded well, and that there were innovative ways of making better use of the human resource base employed within the authority. In effect, a mandate for change emerged from this first step towards the implementation of a strategic architecture, one that has now fed into the development of many more integrating processes in respect of service design. Kiosks have been installed across the council boundaries, delivering information and in some cases facilitating payment of local taxes. BCC-administered buildings and services, particularly the public library service, have been redefined in respect of their role as community assets, with some movement towards treating them as the 'high street' operating hub of the council with full electronic access to a wide range of council services.

The Mobile Office Strategy is a further case in point, and has important linkages to issues around not only IM but also KM. Here, field workers are linked electronically to their office base and – perhaps more critically – to the call centre, using portable computers, modems and mobile telephones, facilitating considerable improvements in response rates and information exchange, and in the emergence of a widespread culture of co-operation and co-ordination which has contributed to a very real sense of working towards the achievement of a truly 'joined-up' approach to service delivery.

It would be wrong, in a brief case study, to give the impression that BCC has achieved considerable ICT-mediated change without encountering any problems. This would be simply unrealistic – it is a large and complex organisation and, as such, any change is unlikely to be achieved without some resistance. However, the reason it is so important, remaining as it does one of only a few such examples observable globally, is that by placing information as opposed to technology at the centre of the change agenda, it has achieved an integration of approach and clarity of operating vision that most public services could be well advised to study as a source of lessons on good practice. Perhaps the most important lesson of all is that BCC now sees itself as being in a position to offer services on behalf of other organisations – the voluntary sector, even other Commonwealth (national) government departments. The argument is that the end-user doesn't care who the service provider is, as long as they can demonstrate that they do it well, with a focus firmly upon quality, reliability and convenience of provision – an argument which is surely of some considerable relevance to public sector policy-makers and strategists.

Chapter 7

Tension and paradox

Issues of information security, ownership, access, liability and openness

The preceding chapters have been intended to provide both general and, where possible, specific guidance on the development of IKM-focused models of public sector operation. We must now move to a critical area of consideration where to seek to make generalisations is both inherently difficult and, in some cases, possibly even dangerous. Issues of information security, freedom of information, data protection, privacy, copyright, intellectual property and the achievement of that somewhat paradoxically viewed aspiration, 'open' government – all these require significant levels of consideration by those planning to modernise or change the way in which public sector structures position themselves to interface within and across government and with the external client or citizen. However, as we shall also discuss, a certain amount of pragmatism and reality are much-needed ingredients in any 'recipe' likely to deliver successful outcomes.

Developing information 'reality'

For the external observer, the apparent contradictions and tensions that are discernible in many major democracies today can appear insoluble, linked as they are to issues of ensuring security of information holdings competing with rhetoric proclaiming commitment to the achievement of more open and transparent ways of providing public services,. As we have already discussed, principles of IKM are underpinned by a commitment to the establishment of an operating culture where internal information-sharing and the exchange of ideas, observations and experience are the norm rather than the exception. Perhaps the most significant catalyst for the growing debate around the competing demands of access and security has been the growth in the adoption and importance of ICTs within government. Technology-enabled or driven change, depending upon the degree of latitude that one allows to permeate discussions in this area, has served to both particularise and magnify a number of issues and concerns which have been discussed for some two centuries.

If we look at the examples of the United States and Sweden, where principles and associated laws providing for the public's right of access to government information have been enshrined within the democratic constitution for two hundred years, we can see that it is possible to govern reasonably successfully within clearly defined parameters for citizen access. However, contrast this with the position of the government of the United Kingdom, where legislation to enable freedom of information to be enacted from a citizen perspective, although much discussed, has as yet failed to reach the statute books. Consider then these two disparate approaches to enshrining some right of access to information within a legislative framework alongside the 1946 declaration of the United Nations, which states: 'freedom of information is a fundamental human right and is the touchstone for all the freedoms to which the United Nations is consecrated' (United Nations 1946: 59(1)).

In an IKM context there can probably be at least two responses to the statement presented above. The first might be an immediate agreement that meaningful improvements in information-intensive methods of delivering public services cannot be realised in the absence of well-constructed legislation, setting out frameworks and parameters for citizen access to information. However, it is possible, although probably controversial, to argue that IKM in government can operate successfully without any such explicit legislation and that issues of information security are, in fact, of rather more importance, particularly those which concern any opportunities for fraud or mismanagement of resources. Perhaps, in balancing the competing claims of these two positions, the most pragmatic position to adopt here is one of information *reality*: almost regardless of whether legislation around access to public sector information holdings exists, this is largely (although, of course, not entirely) a societal issue, and as such is likely to be of greatest concern to politicians and citizen lobbying groups. Senior public sector managers alive to the potential afforded by the adoption of IKM principles have a duty to be, above all else, realists in their dealings around information access and security and the tensions that may exist between the two.

Such an approach, based upon information reality and pragmatism, has to achieve a balance between the societal concerns in the present dominant operational culture of the public sector, whereby many politicians champion not only 'better government', but also 'open government': the latter, as Chapman and Hunt argue,

> refers to various issues associated with government secrecy. It refers to the ability of the public in a democracy to hold the government fully accountable for its actions and to assess the validity of actions taken. It also refers to the rights of individual citizens in relation to information about them held in public organisations.
>
> (Chapman and Hunt 1987: 11)

Such a definition is something beyond 'simply' freedom of information; it represents a development in the notions of accountability that underpin our commonly understood frameworks of democratic principle. The balance, however, must be achieved by IKM strategists between the open government position, which some cynics describe as representing a contradiction in terms in itself, and a workable way of moving forward the efficiency and effectiveness of public services; this involves a critical realisation that such a position of access and accountability will be, to a large degree and almost in spite of any legislation affected, dependent upon the way in which the public sector understands and utilises its information assets. Democratising and making accessible a fragmented and largely unstructured mass of data and information is likely to benefit, or indeed interest, only a minority of society, whereas the challenges and opportunities associated with IKM are potentially far greater in respect of developing a culture of accountability for information holdings within the public sector.

Thus, although IKM-focused policy and strategy development must demonstrate cognisance of both legislation and political inclination, it should not necessarily use this as a starting point for effecting major change. Rather, the issues of greatest immediate concern may well be the lack of standardisation across constituent parts of the public sector and the inhibiting effect of this upon opportunities for engendering a culture, attitude and style of working which make internal co-operation and collaboration possible while leveraging the end-user experience of public service interface. It could be argued that the adoption of such an approach will contribute more to the achievement of a truly open public sector structure than a more obvious legislative focus upon issues around freedom of information, which may provide the illusion of enhanced access to public services without any real mechanism for doing so.

Standardisation across government

As has been discussed above, legislation in respect of citizen access to information can only ever achieve partial improvements in any public sector reform or modernising agenda. Curious and even extreme anomalies exist between countries. Perhaps one of the best examples comes from the European Union: here, citizens denied access to EU information in one country, where regulation rather than freedom is the dominant practice in respect of information holdings, may access it through channels in another, more liberal member country. As a result, it is not surprising that there is often a public sense of frustration at the lack of clarity or coherence that exists not only across governments but also often within them. Addressing such disparities offers key opportunities for effecting real and qualitative improvements in the citizen experience of interfacing with strands of public sector operation. However, effecting this change will require considerable determination on the part of IKM leaders, for in a real sense the challenge is not just to set about creating a new operating culture but, perhaps much more significantly, to break through the legacies of past practice. These have led to individual systems and methodologies developing within and across different public sector operating strands which might, if one were of a cynical disposition, be viewed as having been designed with the intention of preventing cross-functional working or logical delivery of front-end services to the citizen as user.

Freedom of information (FOI) and IKM

If realism and pragmatism are the requisite approaches for working to enact an IKM approach within the public sector, they must, of course, be informed by any existing relevant legislation. As has been outlined previously, the United States and Sweden have been in the vanguard of ensuring that citizens have a clearly defined right to access information produced by their public sector – albeit with some caveats that relate to issues of national competition, individual privacy and security and defence. Such approaches have been influential, as other countries have moved to adopt legislation in this area: for example, in perhaps the most recent example of a major piece of FOI legislation, that executed by the government of the Republic of Ireland in 1997, it is clearly articulated that the primary objectives are:

> An Act to enable members of the public to obtain access, to the greatest extent possible, consistent with the public interest and the right to privacy, to information in the possession of public bodies and to enable persons to have personal information relating to them in the possession of such bodies corrected and, accordingly, to provide for a right of access to records held by such bodies, for necessary exceptions to that right and for assistance to persons to enable them to exercise it, to provide for the independent review both of decisions of such bodies relating to that right and of the operation of this Act generally (including the proceedings of such bodies pursuant to this Act) and for those purposes, to provide for the establishment of the Office of Information commissioner and to define its functions, to provide for the publication by such bodies of certain information about them relevant to the purposes of this Act, to amend the Official Secrets Act, 1963, and to provide for related matters.
>
> (Ireland, Department of Finance 1997: 3)

What it is critical to record here, in relation to the way in which the public sector views its information and knowledge holdings, is the potential impact that articulation of rights of access may have upon the operating culture of public services. In the relatively recent example of Ireland, the scope and scale of the change upon all types of public service organisation has been acknowledged through compulsory briefings for all employees upon both the remit and potential impact of FOI legislation upon their work. Likewise, citizen education and communication has proved to be a second crucial element in giving life to the Act for, after all, if only a small interested elite of your population actually understand the implications of a move towards providing greater access to public sector information holdings, then the overall effect is likely to be minimal.

So it may be argued that, beyond simply drafting legislation, there are linked imperatives to educate both public service employees and users as to the rights, responsibilities and limitations represented by FOI legislation. In terms of IKM, this can undoubtedly serve as a useful building block on the road to achieving an open and sharing culture across tiers of public service. Potentially, such ongoing education can serve to highlight the notion of information as a commodity, an 'asset' as we have discussed previously, something which requires the same, if not greater, care in its management as matters of finance or other resources. Thus, it can legitimately be envisaged that there are important organisational cultural gains to be made from moving to a position where freedom of information is part of the way that government is structured to do business with its citizens, and indeed can be held more widely accountable for its actions and behaviour.

However, it would be wrong to think of FOI legislation as representing some universal panacea for ensuring the achievement of IKM-focused public services, for the long-standing examples of access cited in Sweden and the United States have not served to effect markedly different modes of operation from those found in a country such as the United Kingdom, which has no such legislation in place. The main gains stemming from FOI, articulated in purely IKM terms, are those previously stated: the development of a culture where information is understood, at least partially, as an asset or commodity, to which the citizen may request access. However, in respect of achieving 'joined-up' or 'open' government, it cannot be said with any real credibility that an emphasis upon freedom of information has served to achieve real structural changes in the way in which public services operate. Indeed, the execution of FOI legislation does little to require that citizens actually have access to any sort of rationalised information holdings. Thus, although a specific query might involve accessing information held by revenue services, benefits agencies and a health department, FOI legislation generally would make no requirement upon public sector structures that access should be seamless: the message is simply that, while access may be ensured, within certain defined limitations, there is no requirement that it should be logical or even necessarily easy for the citizen. Thus, there is a lingering sense, as we shall explore in Chapter 8, that the absence of well-thought-out IKM principles can actually serve to exclude all but the most articulate citizen from engaging with public services in a way which is meaningful and addresses their specific needs.

Thus it is inherently inaccurate to posit an argument that sees the central requirement of achieving new and better modes of delivering services to citizens as necessarily being the enshrining of access to information within legislation of rights. As a building block and a component, such an approach is certainly beneficial, for it does serve to set clear parameters for what should and can be accessed within the public domain. However, what no FOI legislation actually addresses is the contribution that opening up access to public service information can serve to make on the way that the public sector is itself structured. Typically, within such legislation there is no suggestion that a better citizen experience of accessing public service information might be gained if individual departments and tiers of government were required and enabled to access and share information across their traditional operating boundaries. Thus, although we may look to the examples of the United States and Sweden as being beacons of long-term constitutional recognition of the rights of the citizen to access information held by their public services, it is not possible to say that either country differs dramatically from others with more recent and emerging commitments in this area with respect to how public service structures operate in relation to one another: indeed, the barriers – both cultural and (increasingly) technological – to logical and integrated service provision remain, and in some instances are becoming increasingly exacerbated.

Thus a key challenge for the IKM strategist is to examine ways in which freedom of information practice and rhetoric can be harnessed to add value to the goal of creating a new way of public sector working. At a purely structural level, as we have discussed in earlier chapters, IKM is reliant for its success upon the development of operating structures and cultures framed by a logic which recognises that exploiting synergies and linkages, underpinned by information and knowledge assets, represents the best way of achieving a 'joined-up' model of public service provision. A key driver in delivering this new model of public sector provision is undoubtedly the desire to create something which is at once more resource-efficient and addresses the citizen experience of interacting with public services. Access to certain types and levels of information, while legitimately held to be a fundamental civil liberty, does not necessarily guarantee that citizens will experience an enhanced level of satisfaction with their public services, nor that they will always clearly understand their rights as set out in law in respect of information held. Thus, in an IKM context, it is important to view issues of FOI within a realistic perspective, and to acknowledge at the outset that they are not particularly close relatives: indeed, to extend the family relationship metaphor, they are perhaps more accurately described as cousins rather than siblings.

Freedom of information is in itself an important and distinct area of study, one which engages passions and principles in a way which it is possible to argue that IKM will never do. However, it may well be right to posit a view that the logical benefits of introducing and embedding a dynamic culture of citizen rights in respect of information holdings can never be fully realised until the model of IKM-driven public services discussed in this text begins to become widely practised. While the existence of legislation may have some beneficial impacts upon the way in which employees order their work, perhaps with a view to later access by the citizen, what it critically does not require of public services is that they impose any citizen-centric logic upon their ways of working. Public sector structures within even the most FOI-friendly nations remain compartmentalised, with little openness and standardisation of approach which might facilitate easier and more meaningful citizen access. It is, therefore, illusory to believe that an emphasis upon ensuring 'freedom' of access to information will deliver public sector structures which can be defined in terms of 'open' government: the latter requires a breadth of structural and internal cultural change which, while certainly enabled to some extent by specific FOI legislation, will be far more reliant for its achievement upon clearly articulated principles of IKM serving to change the way that public services fundamentally create, exchange and share information-based services and ultimately make them available to the citizen.

Data protection and privacy legislation

A global overview of legislation in the area of data protection and personal rights to privacy reveals a plethora of Acts and Directives, most of which have emerged since the 1970s. These seek to enshrine in law principles protecting the individual's rights over data and information about them obtained and held by third parties and, in the case of data protection specifically, primarily stored electronically. Legislation typically covers all sectors, although there may be permitted caveats, or opportunities for permission to be gained to step outside the standard principles of the law if a case can be made for a 'greater public good' being achieved by compromising the integrity of data protection or privacy rights for particular individuals.

Consideration of the Canadian-based Access to Justice Network, which is available via the World Wide Web (http://www.acjnet.org/resource/primary.html), is an excellent source with which to begin any attempt at an international overview of practice in this area. For not only does it address specific pieces of legislation, as well as emerging influential reports and draft documents, on a country-by-country basis, but it also acknowledges and reflects upon the increasing need to work within international agreements and directives – for example, the influential European Union's Directive on Data Protection, enacted in 1996.

Typically, much data protection legislation can be described in terms outlined by the UK's Data Protection Registrar, who explains that:

> The Data Protection Act (1998) is concerned with 'Personal Data' (this is information about living identifiable individuals. This need not be particularly sensitive information, and can be as little as name and address) which is 'automatically processed'. It works in two ways, giving individuals certain rights whilst requiring those who record and use personal information on computer to be open about that use and to follow sound and proper practices.
>
> (Data Protection Registrar 1999: 3)

To this end, what typically may happen is that organisations, be they in the public or private sector, must register the type and scale of information holdings that they maintain, and agree to abide by established modes of practice in respect of passing on that information to third parties and to ensure a right of citizen access to check the accuracy of the holdings.

Within a public sector IKM context, issues of data protection and privacy can be perceived to present significant barriers to the establishment of more open and cross-boundary modes of service design and delivery. Furthermore, it is important to question the extent to which the citizen feels concern around matters of privacy; indeed, in outlining the results of twenty-two major studies into the specific issue of 'how concerned are you about your privacy?', Westin revealed that 85 per cent of respondents indicated some level of concern, while of these 55 per cent stated that they were 'very concerned' (Westin 1996). However, it is possible to argue that rather than representing a barrier to the achievement of new modes of service structuring and delivery in the public sector, such concerns can be successfully input into the development of IKM policies and strategies, providing operating guidelines and parameters which serve as both a check, and where necessary, a brake upon the scale of appropriate information and knowledge sharing that it is possible to attain. If an underpinning goal of IKM in the public sector can be said to be the achievement of more user-friendly, coherent and relevant modes of providing information and services to citizens, then this must certainly be supported by a sense of responsibility and respect for the integrity of the resource that is being managed. If this is lost sight of, both in planning and in execution, then not surprisingly issues of suspicion, even alarm, may be generated, and these may serve to negate many or even all of the benefits sought in moves towards a more IKM-efficient mode of public service.

However, to represent issues of citizen privacy and data protection as being in themselves sufficient reason for halting any progress towards a more rational and user-friendly mode of public sector operation, as some observers have done, is to overstate the extent to which such concerns may produce barriers to change. Properly focused IKM-driven models for re-examining the way in which tiers and strata of public service provision operate represent in themselves no significant threat to either the legal or the ethical status of the treatment of data and information held on citizens by their governments – unless, that is, there is insufficient consideration given to these critical areas. For if a focus upon the legal and ethical dimensions of information-sharing, privacy, access and exploitation is largely absent, then, quite legitimately, issues of concern and public accountability should be raised.

Perhaps one of the best ways of learning how to incorporate sensitivity for issues around data protection, ethical standards of use and privacy into an articulated policy on changing the way in which a public service harnesses and utilises its IKM assets, is to consider controversial Icelandic proposals around health information. Posited internally as a way of supporting health service planning and investment strategy, proposals centre around the creation of a centralised electronic database, containing the detailed medical records, including genetic and other personal data, benefits records and information on prescribed pharmaceutical products, relating to all Icelanders, to be leased for a considerable fee to a commercial company. It is held that, for reasons of historical development, the national population may serve to provide valuable generalisable commercial data on genetic mutation as it relates to major global diseases such as cancer. The proposal, known as the 'Decode Project', has generated international debate and, in some cases, positive censure of the Icelandic proposal. There are concerns that it is seeking to maximise opportunities gained through information-sharing to an unacceptable extent, whereby individual citizens' rights of personal privacy might be compromised, in the absence of adequate safeguards, for what can ultimately be characterised as commercial gain. These views were clearly articulated at the International Conference on Data Protection, held in September 1998 and attended by Data Protection Commissioners of European Union and other European countries, who stressed the importance of the Icelandic government acknowledging that:

> The principle of free and informed consent of the person concerned to the storage and further processing of his or her data must be fully respected. The data subject must also be given the right to withdraw from the base once his or her data have been entered. Exemption from these principles would only be acceptable for exceptional reasons and with adequate safeguards for the correct use of data.
>
> The definition of 'personal data' must be explicitly clear and the method of securing anonymity must be effective. In a country with a relatively small population information or genetics data is likely to indicate biological lineage and to reveal identities of persons concerned. The use of a code to replace identifiers is in any case not sufficient to

secure anonymity ... They [the Data Protection Commissioners] express their serious concern about the matter and recommend the Icelandic authorities to reconsider the project in the light of fundamental principles laid down in the European Convention on Human Rights, the Council of Europe Convention 108 on Data Protection and Recommendation (97)5 on medical data, and the EC Directive 95/46 on the protection of personal data.

(Data Protection Registrar 1999: 5)

Of course, it is true to say that issues of personal information relating to health are always likely to be regarded as having particularly sensitive connotations when considered in respect of the benefits which may be gained by opening up opportunities for pooling or sharing the holdings of a number of stakeholding groups. However, to assume the pragmatic position advocated at the outset of this chapter would be to have adopted, from inception of the 'Decode' proposals, far more focused parameters of use than those currently articulated by the Icelandic proposals, which appear designed almost specifically with the intent of inviting the sort of criticism and concern that we have considered above. Where there is an intention to use IKM principles, as is being posited here, to inform government planning and decision-making, the objectives and inbuilt safeguards protecting the individual and society more generally must be clearly articulated. Central to the dilemma posed by the proposals in Iceland is the issue of having identified all of the theoretical benefits of IKM without any apparent acknowledgement of the 'costs' accruing from ignoring the citizen almost completely, as being a stakeholder with any legitimate right of concern over the way in which sensitive personal information might be utilised by their government and, through their leasing arrangement, commercial sector third parties such as pharmaceutical firms. The lesson here is surely that properly constructed data protection and privacy legislation should not be viewed as an obstacle to the achievement of public sector IKM, but rather as serving to provide a helpful parameter which can serve to build citizen confidence in the inherent integrity of the way in which governments regard their role as guardians, rather than owners, of information assets.

Such discussion around data protection, privacy legislation and related guidelines should also be framed within a more general public sector requirement: namely, that all governments should operate at a base level of ethical practice with regard to the way in which they utilise any information of which they are custodian, particularly that which relates to individual citizens. Increasingly within all types of organisations, there is greater focus upon the need to build in an ethical dimension to both policy and strategy development; this should fundamentally challenge all proposals in the IKM area, asking not only, 'Will this enhance the way that we do business, and does it fall within the bounds of extant and emerging legislation?' but also,

'Can it be said to represent ethical and accountable behaviour measured against identified norms or guidelines?'

Issues of ownership: copyright and intellectual property in the IKM environment

A focus upon the legal environment framing concepts of information and knowledge ownership, whether it is expressed in something as tangible as a patent for a specified product or copyright covering a volume of poetry, or something as abstract as an 'idea' posted on a web page, does immediately throw up some questions concerning how it can best be addressed in a specifically public sector setting. Covered by national laws and international conventions and treaties, most notably the Berne Convention of 1988 covering issues of copyright and the WIPO (World Intellectual Property Organization) Treaty of 1996, such agreements set out base-level recommendations that signatories must adopt as a minimum level of national protection for tangible and intangible asset protection, while allowing for local variations and additions to legislation to take account of particular national requirements.

Copyright legislation, although variously applied across nations, could be said to represent an area of some concern in certain public sector operating environments, when it may find itself serving as a barrier to the opening up and sharing of information holdings, both across public sector bodies and with other organisations or individuals who may be key stakeholders. Of course, while it is true to say that governments must accept and maintain high levels of responsibility for protecting their information products and the integrity of their publications, an over-zealous and over-protectionist interpretation of copyright legislation can serve to make the achievement of IKM-friendly structures infinitely more difficult to realise.

It can be argued that approaches to copyright within the public sector are very likely to mirror internal perceptions and operating culture around the degree of freedom and openness that should be encouraged in public service operations. While it is, of course, understandable that the public sector should protect certain of its assets from unscrupulous exploitation and possible corruption through appropriate use of copyright conventions, questions should be asked as to whether re-evaluation of wholesale copyright applications across the public sector might result in something more appropriate to much of the 'documentation' that the government produces.

In moving to consider issues around intellectual property, Torremans and Holyoak provide some useful guidance on the degree of synergy which is evident in the blurring of definition in relation to the concept of copyright:

> When we refer to intellectual property rights, we do not wish to make the distinction between the industrial intellectual property rights, such

as patents and trade marks, and artistic intellectual property rights, such as copyright. We think this distinction is no longer valid as copyright is now used in such a flexible way, for example to protect computer programs, that it can no longer be called an exclusively artistic right. The same concepts underlie each type of intellectual property. A strong form of unity exists between all types of intellectual property and the common law concepts in use in this area.

(Torremans and Holyoak 1998: 5–6)

Aside from concerns to protect internally 'owned' intellectual property rights, a key concern for public sector organisations must be their responsibility to respect the rights of other parties with whom they contract. Typically, concerns in this area have arisen out of poorly articulated and understood contractual arrangements with commercial or quasi-commercial agency status parties, who have provided a product or who manage a service on behalf of a public sector department. For example, although largely absent from any formal discussion in the literature, there have certainly been incidents where ICT providers have felt that public services have compromised or breached their intellectual property rights, through permitting competitor access to tailor-made programs and packages. Of course, it may be argued that this becomes almost inevitable in a climate where public sector contracting remains fragmented and where there is increasing pressure to enact methodologies to enable cross-functional sharing of information. The implications of such developments are potentially enormous and must, at the very least, inform any intention to roll out cross- or even sometimes inter-departmental collaborations.

Information security

Aside from specifically legal and ethical concerns around issues of access to and protection of the public sector information and knowledge base, operational issues of security must also be recognised as a central plank in building a workable case for increasing and improving citizen access to public services. As we have seen in discussions around FOI and copyright particularly, there has been something of a tendency in the public sector to emphasise the degree of security which needs to be attached to information use and exchange. However, where what might be described as a 'blanket' approach applies, in which almost everything is held to be in need of securing for the public good, some important questions need to be asked around the extent to which enhanced service levels based upon appropriate and logical citizen access to services can be achieved. Vareljs argues that such blanket approaches are wholly inappropriate in any organisation, and that there needs to be a critical review of operations which, in respect of information holdings, questions:

- the degree of sensitivity of information;
- the hierarchy of applications to which security arrangements should apply;
- the costs and benefits of such applications.

(Vareljs 1996: 26)

If we consider first the way in which information is classified and the impact that the assignment of such a classification may have upon use, it is, of course, apparent that widely differing degrees of sensitivity will be attached to holdings within the public sector generally. Most problematic is the fact that only rarely are there clearly articulated criteria by which information sensitivity is formally assigned, leaving inherent dangers that innate human conservatism may result in far too much being deemed to be for restricted access, both internally and externally. While it is fair to say that legal implications around data protection and official secrets, or other national security legislation, are commonly fed into some formal categorisation of information held, too often they are cited as a reason for over-classifying and therefore restricting the use of the information itself.

Such observations in an IKM context illustrate, if further illustration were needed, that operational cultures more than any other factor present the greatest barrier to achieving a more effective mode of public service. Vision, determination and education would seem to be the essential ingredients required to move forward a radical and far-reaching review of how information sensitivity is classified, moving from a predominant model which, it can be argued, sees the public good as best protected by an emphasis upon blanket security arrangements and protocols, to one which emphasises access, underpinned by appropriate levels of security. To move this agenda forward will require all of the leadership skills previously referred to, as well as an emphasis upon educating the public sector employee in the way in which information sensitivity is classified.

Linked to this overarching issue of information security classification is the need to simultaneously question the critical applications to which issues of security must be applied. The 'blanket' approach referred to previously, which sees all strands of operation and all tiers of public service provision as potentially in need of security applications, is a fundamentally negative one. In an IKM environment, the emphasis should instead be upon identifying which applications and services have low or negligible security implications, and removing from them any barriers to more efficient and effective operation. Instead of argument being constructed upon a principle which requires that a case should be made for lowering security classification, the emphasis should instead be upon requiring that a persuasive reason can be put forward for retaining or increasing levels of information security. Such a repositioning of public sector ethos around issues of access and security represents a considerable cultural shift in its own right, but it is a shift that is critical to the achievement of any of the benefits posited for adopting an IKM focus in the public sector. Therefore, alongside an evaluation and rationalisation of existing modes of information security classification, it should also be required that all applications be audited against criteria constructed to reflect the relative value of processes to effecting both internal and external service enhancement.

The final component of this model for reviewing information security emphasises the requirement that consideration of both costs and benefits should be incorporated into any decision-making equation. Such costs and associated benefits, while having direct resource and financial implications, also involve consideration of factors which might be best termed as 'philosophical considerations', at least in the first instance. Most importantly, the question that must be asked is what, if any, are the implications of the wide-scale reduction of levels of security relating to information holdings: are there associated costs in respect of maintaining the inherent integrity of public sector operations? Alongside this question must of course be set the question of what benefits might possibly accrue from 'opening up' information holdings, enabling them to be used in innovative and access-oriented ways.

Debate generated by the asking of such questions will typically involve politicians, public sector employees, usually working at a senior level, and often lawyers with a specialism in the various areas discussed in this chapter. Of particular interest in an emerging global context is the further cost/benefit element associated with issues of legal admissibility of information exchanges, both internal to the public sector and in exchange with citizens and other parties. The danger, of course, in opening up such a debate is that issues of security around information held by the public sector, and in particular involving matters pertaining to the individual citizen, can quite properly raise considerable degrees of concern, effectively polarising issues of security and access, which may serve to overwhelm any arguments around achieving a new and more citizen-centric mode of public governance.

However legitimate concerns may be concerning the potential 'costs' of reviewing security arrangements associated with information holdings in order to achieve a 'benefit' of new modes of delivering public services, channels for overcoming these concerns should be built into any discussion. Issues of information security are not new, nor are they unique to the public sector, and it is in the practice of other service-oriented organisations that pointers to modes of achieving a workable balance between information security and access may be achieved. Increasingly, as we have previously discussed, new models of public service delivery, using as their templates practice in other sectors, are introducing a range of technologies to enhance the user experience of access to both information and services. However, moving into an environment whereby the end-user either directly, or in a mediated forum, has access to information holdings from something which might be described as a 'one-stop shop' does raise major issues around how the security of information can be guaranteed, especially in an environment where, as Vareljs argues: 'an individual intent on causing damage could begin in the morning and have a DUI (Driving Under the Influence) charge on your driver's license by the afternoon' (Vareljs 1996: 25).

Into this 'brave new world' of technology-mediated information provision and service delivery must therefore be introduced the need to consider appropriate security measures which can serve to protect the integrity of public sector ICT holdings. Such applications will not, of course, be without associated costs, which in resource terms are both ongoing and potentially substantial; however, it may be argued that without them, concerns around information security, articulated internally and serving as a potential barrier to the enactment of change agenda, and the critical issue of building and maintaining citizen confidence in new modes of working, will never be successfully addressed.

To consider, then, some of the established and emerging tools for providing required levels of security in a public sector context. Those discussed here have a common underpinning theme: they are concerned with ensuring the authentication of the user, thus attempting to provide a security framework whereby hierarchies or classes of information identified as requiring a level of security limiting them to access by identified individuals, be they internal or external to the organisation, are protected by a range of hardware and software applications. To this end, as an external citizen seeking to enter or check personal revenue data via an Internet application, one might find that certain authentication procedures would be followed prior to access being permitted.

Vareljs discusses a number of the established and emerging tools which could reasonably be deployed in a public sector setting. The first, and perhaps most commonly used, a 'firewall', already has considerable public sector take-up; indeed, such security measures underpin the fast-expanding Government Secure Intranet (GSI) project, which is promoting the internal exchange of information within the UK public sector. Defined as a 'powerful network security tool consisting of hardware and software that allow your organisation access to Internet resources whilst prohibiting unwanted incursions from the Internet into your organisation' (Vareljs 1996: 26), a firewall is also a flexible security tool which can be applied selectively, if so desired, allowing easy external access to areas where this is held not to be problematic or indeed is seen as positively desirable, while permitting security and protection to be provided to other more sensitive areas of operation.

A further and increasingly sophisticated security tool in the electronic information environment is that of encryption, which may be described as a process or tool-kit which:

keeps information transmitted via a communications link safe from unauthorized access and tampering. The encryption process involves converting the original message (plaintext) into unreadable form (ciphertext) through the use of an encoding algorithm by the authorized sender. When the resulting ciphertext is sent across the network, would-be eavesdroppers using taps and network analyzers can collect the ciphertext but cannot unscramble the material. Decryption occurs when the intended recipient reconverts the ciphertext back to the original plaintext with the use of a key. A key is a string of digital information allowing users to encode or decode a message.

(Vareljs 1996: 28)

In moving forward the goal of increasing citizen access to information holdings and services, there has been considerable focus upon taking issues of authentication beyond firewall and encryption devices. Thus we have seen the concept of the 'electronic signature' gaining a considerable momentum, particularly among those within the public sector who view technology-mediated change as being the most likely vehicle for delivering enhanced service provision. Whether this is likely to result in widespread adoption of smartcard applications or voice-recognition security tools – or in the most sophisticated 'biometric' approach thus far deployed, individual cornea patterns – is something which remains more discussed than actioned. However, what does seem clear is that, in order to ensure public confidence and provide proper security and governance policies for information holdings, such issues will require considerable strategic focus and associated investment.

Information security: the question of responsibility

The intention of this chapter, as stated at the outset, was primarily to raise issues of general concern and to position them within an operational framework which acknowledged the requirement to ensure that due attention was paid to relevant national – and in some cases international – legislation. However, beyond adherence to specific legal requirements, there is a further imperative which must be addressed at senior levels within all organisations: the need for overarching responsibility and accountability for information security to be clearly recognised and assigned at an appropriate level of seniority. The implications here for the public sector are enormous, with the general problem of fragmented approaches to practice in service design and delivery being replicated in the various approaches to the setting of protocols for ensuring the protection of information and knowledge assets. A move towards the creation of IKM-enabled modes of working, with a considerably enhanced emphasis upon the sharing of such assets, should point to the need for the public sector to address issues of security, balanced against particular access goals. At an overarching strategic level, this would involve the development of security measures and approaches which could be deployed across most tiers of public sector operation.

It is important to note that an absence of sufficient organisational focus upon the issue of information and knowledge security is not unique to the public sector; in the commercial sector, issues of negligence and neglect have been emphasised by the findings of the 1998 *Information Security Survey*, which surveyed a thousand organisations in the United Kingdom and Ireland, each with an annual turnover of more than £10 million. Taking the report's definition of information security provides a useful initial focus for those interested in public sector applications: 'information security is defined as the practices and procedures which ensure that information, generally held in electronic format, is safeguarded from unauthorised access, modification or accidental change and is readily available to authorised users on request' (*Information Security Survey* 1998: 1). Importantly, here we have the key issues of security and access shown to be in reality two aspects of IKM, so closely entwined that they might be said to represent two sides of the same coin.

The *Information Security Survey* identified, as part of its analysis of data returned, a number of major areas of concern, at least some of which must be held to be generalisable across the public sector; key among them: that aspects of 'electronic commerce' represent a major security threat; that security offences are going undetected; that recovery plans remain untested; and that, more generally, security policies are inadequate (*Information Security Survey* 1998: 1).

In a public sector context, electronic commerce – that is, transactions involving some movement of a resource, usually financial, mediated by an ICT tool – are gaining increasing penetration, and this is likely to grow as a momentum around modernising government takes hold. However, the experience of the commercial sector in respect of the adoption of electronic commerce contains at least some cautionary warnings:

> The single most important business issue in terms of its likely impact on security was considered to be Electronic Commerce … 70 per cent of organisations used the Internet, almost double the figure from the previous survey in 1996. Yet of those organisations using the Internet, over three quarters had not tested the security of their Internet site and less than half of users and intended users had procedures covering the use of the Internet. A third of Internet users had systems which do not provide security violation reporting or did not review it … these risks and exposures are not being properly managed because organisations either do not fully understand them or cannot visualise their impact.
>
> (*Information Security Survey* 1998: 1)

To contextualise the concerns articulated here within a public administration model, it is useful to revisit the examples extant in Australia, discussed in earlier chapters with particular reference to the Centrelink model and the Brisbane call centre, which may be defined generically as representing 'single entry points' to public services. In an important report on the implications of enhancing the levels of information-sharing within the public sector, the ICA, focusing upon the example of Centrelink, revealed that it typically received 1.6 million Internet enquiries per year; it was moving to a position of electronic transfer of benefits mediated by Internet technology, and discussed the need to take on board important security implications around such developments:

> For full functionality of the single entry point in an Internet environment, a range of security and legal issues need to be addressed and strategies for handling these issues are being developed. The legislative framework, data security and integrity, user authentication, privacy protection and legal liabilities are relevant issues, and will need to be decided upon ... Solutions to a number of technical difficulties associated with the Internet are currently being developed by the private sector and will need to be taken into account. For example, private sector organisations are developing facilities for secure electronic payments across the Internet and are developing commercial signature products (notwithstanding the lack of formal accreditation frameworks or laws concerning digital signatures).
>
> (ICA 1998a: 25)

Importantly, what we see here is acknowledgement of the fact that issues around information security are not unique to public administration and that there must be considerable scope for learning from, and indeed benchmarking against, developing best practice, particularly that emerging from service sector businesses which have realised the value of their information assets to profitability and longer-term growth.

Worryingly, the *Information Security Survey* reveals a lack of awareness among a majority of respondents around the potential threats represented by security breaches:

> Only half of all organisations carry out formal reporting of security incidents and only half of these take action against offenders. In the absence of proper security, organisations are more dependent on users' awareness ... Yet security saves money! Many companies pay three times over for insecurity. Losses are suffered through a security failure; costs are incurred recovering from the incident; followed by more costs to secure systems and prevent further failure. Our survey identified that

there is direct financial benefit from good security and indirect savings as well.

(Information Security Survey 1998: 2)

Once more, it is easy to see that such observations are likely to be generalisable across public sector practice. If a typical model around security can be characterised as reactive, then there is much in suggesting that it may not simply be logical to move away from this position and to take a far more pro-active stance in respect of security, allowing far greater focus on achieving an integrated and effective model of practice. Such a rational and resource-efficient perspective could reasonably be regarded as something for which a senior-level IKM strategist might conceivably wish to assimilate responsibility, within their broader remit for effecting change.

In respect of guaranteeing and testing the robustness of information held, the Survey reports that far too many recovery plans remain untested:

Organisations can only rely on plans if they know they will work. A plan which has not been tested is unpredictable and cannot be relied upon when needed. Although this survey revealed a mild increase in organisations' formulation of recovery plans, 71 per cent of all organisations had never tested their plan.

(Information Security Survey 1998: 2)

Typically, public sector organisations hold disaster plans and routinely back up electronically held information assets. However, what is clearly articulated in the *Information Security Survey* is for all organisations to think through the implications of various disaster and failure scenarios with some degree of care, and to have in place actionable and workable plans for addressing or remedying issues around information failure within clearly defined time scales – all of which should, of course, be tested regularly, to ensure that they remain appropriate and to take note of organisational changes which might have a significant impact upon an established recovery plan.

Liability and responsibility in public sector information provision

An emerging area of importance, when considering potential legal frameworks for developing IKM approaches in the public sector, is the question of liability in respect of outcomes of information supplied to end-users, be they organisations or individuals. In an increasingly litigious society, governments have to consider very carefully the parameters and contexts within which they take responsibility for the outcomes of information, particularly where it can be construed as advice which they send out into public fora.

A particularly interesting example of developments in this area surrounds the creation in the UK of a national health service initiative, NHS Direct. This is, in essence, a call centre operation, staffed by health care professionals, from which the public are encouraged to solicit advice and guidance rather than immediately contacting general practitioners or emergency services. As is common practice in other sectors, all telephone conversations will be recorded, but it remains to be seen how the first cases of misdiagnosis or misunderstanding on the part of adviser or client will be viewed, in respect of the attribution of liability in instances where something has gone wrong.

The issue of responsibility and liability is an appropriate place at which to bring discussion of information ownership, access and security to a close, for it provides an interesting conceptual convergence with issues of IKM more generally. Without assignment and acceptance of responsibility at the most senior level for the management of information and knowledge assets, what emerges is a patchwork of practice which, in a public sector context, will act to constrain any wider intentions to develop services based upon principles of integration and sharing. This assignment of responsibility, together with a clearly set out framework of protocols relating to issues of access, ownership and security, must then be owned much more widely. At present, practice would suggest that there is acknowledgement that *somebody* ought to be providing this overarching leadership; in practice, however, it could be *anybody*, for it is not fully recognised as being a key strategic and operational responsibility, and in effect possibly *nobody* has a clear view of exactly what is happening, which of course impacts upon *everybody*, be they internal or external users.

Allocating overarching responsibility in this area, within the *realistic* framework outlined at the beginning of this chapter, and ensuring that there is co-ordination and collaboration must therefore be seen as a key public sector challenge if the benefits of IKM are to be realised.

Chapter 8

IKM as a tool of social inclusion

In the political rhetoric of the closing years of the twentieth century, the terms 'social inclusion' and 'social exclusion' must rank among those most often cited by those setting out priorities for government and, through it, for the delivery of public services. The theme of this book has, of course, been to explore the potential offered by adopting appropriate IKM strategies within a public sector operating context, on the basis that such a refocusing of organisational cultures and work practices are, in themselves, capable of delivering *better* public services. However, what should not be ignored, among the more traditionally constructed cost/benefit scenarios related to the changes proposed, is that moves towards the achievement of a public sector underpinned by IKM principles could potentially exacerbate 'exclusion' among some strands of society, or, more positively, act to counter this and promote an agenda of 'inclusion', capable of a tangible and positive impact upon society. The apparent contradictions outlined here reflect the inherent dilemma associated with the adoption of IKM: when it is properly thought out it can represent a major and beneficial *opportunity* for change, but the reverse of the IKM coin is that ill-considered and inadequately piloted change represents the *threat* of making things worse within this context, potentially even exacerbating exclusion.

Essentially, social inclusion is about the citizen, and a recognition that all citizens, for reasons of age, economic profile, employment status, education, location or health, to name only the most common factors of potential disadvantage, cannot be held to be a homogeneous mass at whom uniform public sector applications must be directed. If we consider the impact of these factors upon use and potential use, it is interesting to reflect upon an often cited principle of marketing theory, the '80/20' model, which suggests that 80 per cent of 'business', in a typical organisation, is generated by only 20 per cent of the potential customer base. Acknowledging that this pattern may well be replicated in a public sector context, formulating an agenda to promote social inclusion should therefore be framed within an articulation of clearly defined segments of the citizen base, for whom the move from exclusion to inclusion might be mediated through the better design and delivery of key public services.

Achieving qualitative improvements in the lives of the most excluded strata of society represents an ambitious and challenging agenda for any administration, and one which requires the highest levels of strategic and operational planning to bring about quantifiable improvements. When we considered some of the issues around the adoption of IKM principles in Chapter 2, it was stated that there were considerable dangers associated with ill-thought-out rhetoric: the 'words are cheap' syndrome, in effect. Such a caution, in respect of issues of exclusion and inclusion, must be treated very seriously, for the fundamental question must be: how do you transform the excluded, those who may perceive themselves to be marginalised by society more generally, into a stratum of the population who *belong*, who *participate* and who are fully integrated into a dynamic model of twenty-first-century society?

Taking an IKM approach, an obvious starting point is to suggest that directly delivered public services, and those agency-based operations delivering services on behalf of the public sector, might through enhanced use of information and knowledge assets be capable of a far better understanding of the ways in which they interact with various segments of their total populations. Use and analysis of such resources, at an early stage in planning and review, should serve to highlight where there are peaks and troughs of activity, where current delivery mechanisms are inadequate or inappropriate and where barriers, both real and reported, are having a detrimental impact upon use.

The challenge of exclusion: the seductive power of ICTs for policy-makers

A theme emerging with some regularity in many of the previous chapters has been that issues around IKM are often obscured through inappropriate focus and over-reliance for 'solutions' upon the capabilities, real or imagined, of information and communications technologies. Thus, for example, in the UK Government's 1999 White Paper, *Modernising Government*, we see a clearly articulated view of the direction in which it is perceived that public services must move:

> We will use new technology to meet the needs of citizens and business, and not trail behind technological developments … Information technology is changing our lives: the way we work, the way we do business, the way we communicate with each other, how we spend our time. New technology offers opportunities and choice. It can give us access to services 24 hours a day, seven days a week. It will make our lives easier.
>
> (Cabinet Office 1999: 45)

However, in the context of exclusion one must ask whether we can assume that using technology as a panacea to cure all the perceived ills of public services will serve to minimise the degree of disenfranchisement experienced by some of the more vulnerable groups within society more generally – will it actually make their 'lives easier'? The danger, of course, in setting out a mandate for driving forward the adoption of ICT solutions within a public sector reengineering dynamic, is that there may be the risk of making matters much worse. As Lievesey-Howarth, himself a senior executive within the ICT industry, argues:

> There is a real possibility that we will create a society of technology 'haves' and 'have nots'. We can disenfranchise millions of people, in fact some will argue that we are in the process of doing just that ... so much is changing ... we must not think of computer-literate people but people-literate computers. The information society can be built around the citizen, rather than the current trend of government building infrastructure around itself. I am talking about a citizen-direct approach, not a government-direct approach. This is a community issue. We need leaders to tell industry what is good and what is bad. Regrettably there are few leaders doing this.
>
> (Lievesey-Howarth 1997: 32–3)

The view articulated here is an important one, particularly in respect of what is said about the need for public sector change to be focused around the needs of the 'citizen', and, within that broad classification, to be capable of acknowledging that *flexibility* in reconceptualising what is meant by public services is at least as important as the need for *innovation*. Within this scenario, the possibilities and opportunities afforded by moving to an IKM-driven organisational culture should become self-evident. If, that is, as has been the view posited within this text, we accept that one of the best ways – perhaps the only real way – for the public sector to move to a position of being essentially a citizen-centric operation is by acknowledging the benefits of learning and sharing, within and between distinct operating units.

Taking a global view of public sector reform in the closing years of the twentieth century, a simple bibliometric exercise, based upon analysing the frequency of reference to certain key terms, leaves one in no doubt that the dominant model is one which eulogises the benefits of a 'government-direct' approach to change. Certainly, within the often dense texts associated with reports and other documents, it is possible to identify that there is an almost blind faith placed in the fact that there must be a relationship between the achievement of 'joined-up' methods of service provision and the enhancement of the citizen experience of use. However, although much reference is made to commercial sector models of practice from which, it is argued, the public sector would be well advised to learn, there is little credible evidence

to support or sustain a position that would suggest that such models automatically deliver benefits for the most marginalised strata of society.

An holistic view of public sector reform cannot simply ignore concerns
around exclusion, yet despite the attendant rhetoric there is a very real
danger that this may in fact be happening. Policies emerging now are
focusing to an ever greater extent on the potential for achieving ICT-enabled
public services; of course, for a majority of citizens, as we have seen, if this
is set within a properly constructed IKM framework there are potential
gains for both the end-user and the organisation. However, there is a real
danger that too much reliance is being placed upon developing single entry,
standardised gateways to public services which can lead to dangerous
assumptions being made about minimum levels of ability and opportunity
to access these services. It may be that, in reality, such new gateways simply
mirror or possibly even exacerbate issues of exclusion that were prevalent in
more traditional methods of delivery; the likelihood is, however, that
without careful thought and planning harnessing in particular the knowledge base of front-line employees, new service access and delivery
mechanisms, while meeting with the approval of a majority of users, will not
serve to rectify any inequalities within previous usage patterns.

Thus, moving to what may be termed a citizen-centric mode of service
design must involve asking some fundamental questions:

• who are our potential customers/users?
• which customer groups use us most intensively?
• which are our most time/resource intensive operations?
• where are we failing?

Asking such questions on a regular basis, and ensuring that they are asked
of stakeholders within the delivery process who can provide meaningful
answers based upon experience of client-interface, demonstrates a significant use of information and knowledge assets and their value to the process
of redefining public services. Simple audit processes around information
flows can serve to provide a useful basis upon which to begin to map key
activities and interactions; tapping into the wider knowledge base of the
organisation is likely to further enrich the opportunities for *learning* where
and how aspects of service may be failing or problematic.

Any attempt to achieve a shift in emphasis from a 'government-direct' to
a 'citizen-direct' approach to public service design and delivery mechanisms
has to be focused firmly on two key issues, and to resolve, wherever possible,
any tensions that may arise between the two. These issues are the need to
provide services which will be accessible and relevant to the majority of
users, and, at the same time, the need to be able to demonstrating relevance
to those who traditionally have felt most excluded or who have experienced
the most difficulty in their interactions with public services. What this

suggests, of course, is that the achievement of *flexibility* is perhaps the key critical success factor in moving forward this concept of inclusive public services. The suggestion that single gateways or 'one-stop' entry points represent the best and in some cases the only way for modern public services to operate, is a questionable proposition within a context of seeking to serve all of a population as opposed to simply a majority – and here, of course, we immediately identify the limitations of seeking to apply private sector change strategies, without significant reformulation, into public sector scenarios.

The mandate for government is to serve the people – not just the majority of the people. Within this context, public sector reform strategies which posit a reliance upon ICTs as the engine of change are guilty of partial and imperfect understanding of their duties and their environment. However, if administrations can be persuaded to take their policy and strategy formulation to a level which places ICTs within the context of being only a possible tool of change and considers instead, how present structures work, and are prepared to utilise and particularly learn from the information and knowledge assets held, then it is likely that what will emerge will be a mixed-methodology mode of service design. Such an approach acknowledges diversity in society; it recognises that for certain groups – perhaps a majority – a technology-mediated gateway such as a call centre or an Internet-based service represents a significant enhancement in the experience and perceptions of citizens. However, it critically also acknowledges that, for what is possibly a minority, such an approach is profoundly disempowering, and that other methods, possibly access to the 'human interface' in local environments, may be the best and only way of ensuring equal access to the services provided.

Thus, refocusing public service methodologies should not be seen as a single-track, 'one size fits all' approach, at least if a key component of the change agenda is not only to achieve more efficient public services but also to prioritise the need for effectiveness and inclusion. In this context, we can clearly see that if IKM issues are neglected in the approach adopted to deliver change, then critical opportunities for developing and delivering appropriate service mechanisms, and for re-working them to ensure continuing levels of appropriateness, will be missed. Critically, the real danger in respect of public sector change agenda emerging today is that too much emphasis is placed upon the 'given' perception, that change is a one-way street where all the traffic is ICT-driven, whereas if we utilise our IKM assets more fully, the reality, of course, is that there is first a need to ask some fundamental questions. This is something which, as Senge *et al.* observe, is far too rare an occurrence in the typical organisation:

'Stop asking so many questions,' many children hear at home. 'Don't give me the question, give me the answer,' many students hear at school.

'I'm not interested in hearing what you don't know ... I want to hear what you do know,' many employees hear at work. The injunction against discovering and asking questions is widespread in today's family, educational and corporate cultures ... Asking questions is essential for coevolving the futures we want rather than being forced to live with the futures we get.

(Senge *et al.* 1999: 506–7)

Asking questions: an IKM challenge

If asking questions and challenging established modes of delivery and behaviour are accepted as valuable learning tools in driving forward the achievement of consistently appropriate forms of public service, then one must ask within what type of framework this can most effectively happen. It could be argued that, almost as a by-product of the emphasis on public sector change, and in close alignment with the inclusion/exclusion agendas of the late twentieth century, it has been increasingly common for consultation with citizens to take place in respect of their experience of public services. A range of consultation methodologies is evident, from the almost ubiquitous focus group approach adopted by the UK government, which sees the use of 'Peoples' Panels' as a tool to legitimise change agenda, through to more traditional surveys, interviews and other market research tools deployed at varying degrees of regularity: for example, monthly in the case of Brisbane City Council.

However, as with any research tool, one must seriously question both the intent and the value of such approaches to consultation. Designing a research framework which seeks to provide genuinely unbiased and representative data to inform service planning is never going to be a straightforward task. The key difficulty, in the context of this chapter particularly, is of course that groups of the total population held to be most 'excluded' may be precisely the most difficult groups from which to access either qualitative or quantitative data. This, and other allied issues and difficulties, underpinned the development of a possible model of good practice for those engaged in exploring change agenda for public services developed by academics based at the University of North London: the 'ACCESS' model, although designed particularly in respect of 'electronic government' applications, is held to be more widely generalisable (Milner 1999: 63–72).

The term 'ACCESS', used both as an acronym (representing A Citizen-Centric Evaluation of electronic Systems and Services) and as a useful badge in its own right, with its associated resonance with citizen involvement and rights and responsibilities more generally, provides a number of useful pointers to key inputs that can help to ameliorate the dangers of exacerbating issues of exclusion. Critically, the approach advocated within this model recognises the dangers associated with over-emphasis upon the value of information gained from the citizen as end-user:

> Asking citizens to adopt an open and creative system of thought in respect of how they might actually like their public services to be designed for use is, it can be argued, at the present time, in practice an almost impossible and marginal value activity. In order to gain any reliable data to lend credibility to changing strategies or new products, governments and vendors alike, when consulting with end-users, almost always resort to using what are essentially 'loaded' questions, where alternative modes of delivery are suggested to participants. This inherently flawed methodology has tended to result in the evaluation of what is presently available, rather than working towards the achievement of the critical breakthrough into analysis of what the citizen *needs*, *wants* and *expects*. What has resulted has been the plethora of pilots and unco-ordinated projects, the real social and economic value of which must be questioned in the absence of rigorous critical evaluation of outcomes.
>
> (Milner 1999: 67)

Taking this perspective and contextualising it to information, to knowledge transformation, within the model of data that has underpinned our approach to the development of a coherent IKM focus in the public sector, questions arise concerning the relative importance of citizen input. If we accept that external end-users of public services should provide some degree of input into the development of a momentum and an agenda for ongoing learning and associated change, we must do so on the basis that the reliability and generalisability of the information flowing in must be carefully considered. This becomes ever more important in a scenario where there are clear articulations around issues of reducing levels of exclusion. How do you consult meaningfully with those groups who are identified as being most disadvantaged? How do you avoid the dangers inherent in moving to a 'government direct' mode of delivery, supported by citizen consultation exercises, where the net effect may be to marginalise still further those who are already 'excluded', or indeed to create new groups who feel disengaged from service delivery by new modes of operation adopted?

Having the authority and awareness to ask such questions must be regarded as an area of leadership pivotal to the effective deployment of IKM policies and strategies throughout the public sector. In practice, much of what IKM deployment is *about* is the idea that learning and improvement can take place only in a culture where there is proper understanding of the relative value of information and knowledge resources. A key task for any strategist working in this area is to remove or at least restrict the degree of blockage or of 'dead ends' associated with the flows of IKM assets into and around an organisation. When considering ambitious reform agenda, there is an inherent danger that the momentum behind the process can obliterate from sight any degree of design or evaluation input from end-users or, possibly even more importantly, from front-line staff. Weighing up, assigning proper value and, where relevant, 'health warnings' to data, information and knowledge flowing into a consultation loop is possibly the single most important role in developing coherent change agenda. Thus, while it is understandable that in publicly available documents there is a strong emphasis upon the importance of citizen consultation:

> If public services are to serve people better, the Government needs to know more about what people want. Rather than imposing solutions we must consult and work with people. That is why we have set up the *People's Panel*: a 5,000 strong nationally representative group – a world first – to tell us what people really think about their public services and our attempts to make them better. The Panel supplements research being carried out by individual parts of government, including local initiatives such as citizens' juries, community fora and focus groups. We will also build in the views of the customers when measuring the progress that Departments are making against their performance targets in their Public Service Agreements.
>
> (Cabinet Office 1999: 25)

Yet, however laudable this may appear, in terms of the IKM resource gained through the process, the dangers of partiality are obvious: and critically, there is no real acknowledgement that different consultation strategies and mechanisms are likely to be required if a true picture of the experiences and service aspirations of all communities is to be taken into account.

Adapting the notion of the information audit into something which maps the life cycle of a key life 'event' or 'episode' may represent a means of 'asking the right questions' that more appropriately works to encompass the views of both majority stakeholders and of smaller, traditionally more excluded groupings. Thus, if we consider Figure 8.1, taken from the UK Government's 1999 White Paper *Modernising Government*, we can see that the various stages attached to a particular scenario within public service provision are represented. The intention, within the context of this particular document, is to demonstrate the potential complexity of engaging in dialogue with public services, and, in particular to make a case that services should *'reflect people's real lives*. Government should be organised so that people don't have to hunt down services by a process of trial and error' (Cabinet Office 1999: 25).

However, when exploring the potential for overcoming pockets of exclusion from society, an argument emerges which suggests that maximum value may not simply be extracted from looking at such scenario-based flows with

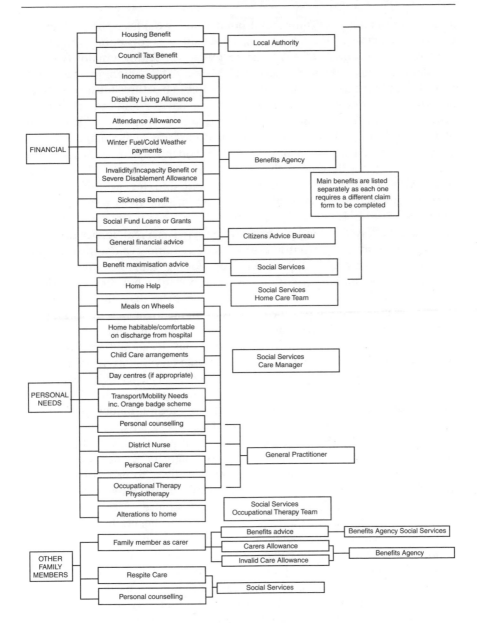

Figure 8.1   Mapping citizen life episodes against extant public sector
structures

Notes: This diagram is for illustration only. The list is not exhaustive and other organisations, friends and family may provide alternative services to those shown.
Crown copyright material is reproduced with the permission of the Controller
of Her Majesty's Stationery Office.

a view to reaching one 'simple' end-point which would see the rationalisation of all or most of the interactions into a single access point, although it
is likely that the benefits of such a process would be felt by a majority of the
population. Rather, a public sector IKM-focused solution to the chaos,
muddle and frustration created by such complex structures must be defined
in terms of its *flexibility* and its *sensitivity*. Single or reduced entry point
systems must be flexible enough to realise that not all of society is made up
of uniform base-level skills, be they defined in terms of language, levels of
literacy or other factors which can create a wider sense of exclusion from
society more generally. One of the key methods, it may be argued, for identifying areas where such flexibility is required and for positing possible
approaches which might be adopted, is to tap into the IKM resource of the
front-line staff. It is they who are most likely to have encountered real
instances where systems and processes have served as a real barrier to use for
some groups. Involving front-line staff in design and evaluation processes
represents a significant opportunity for adding tangible value to the
outcomes of consultation, particularly in respect of what they can add to
the observation of experience by certain groups who may, in service usage
terms at least, be operating at the margins of an inclusive view of society.

Building in sensitivity to consultation and evaluation strategies should be
regarded as so fundamentally important that it should require little
emphasis here. However, this is not to ignore the fact that exercises in infor-
mation- and knowledge-gathering from citizens, as end-users, can serve
effectively to exclude important, and for some groups, critical areas of
concern from planning processes, such as those around literacy, perhaps, or
some impairment of sight, hearing, or language ability. Just as service
delivery informed by IKM resources must be sufficiently flexible to respond
meaningfully to the needs of particular, non-majority segments of society,
so too must such services demonstrate their sensitivity to particular needs if
the intention is both to move to a model of service design and delivery
which will promote inclusiveness, and to use this more widely as a tool for
effecting improvements in the lives of citizens who generally have greatest
difficulty in engaging with public services. In this instance, it is likely that
exploring methodologies for engaging in dialogue with other agencies, such
as voluntary bodies and community groups, may provide a useful input into
the IKM resource base. It must be recognised that other, particularly locally
based, groups may be gateways to a quality and quantity of relevant information and an expertise base that no amount of People's Panels or other
market research can provide.

Information for Health: a UK case study in IKM strategy and its likely impact on social exclusion

When considering, in an operational scenario, the way in which IKM principles are emerging as key drivers of organisational change, and in particular the way in which they converge with issues around overcoming aspects of social exclusion, it is helpful to consider the work beginning to unfold in the United Kingdom's National Health Service (NHS) under the badge of *Information for Health*. Launched in 1998, the strategy document articulates at the outset its underpinning aims:

> The purpose of this information strategy is to ensure that information is used to help patients receive the best possible care. The strategy will enable NHS professionals to have the information they need both to provide that care and to play their part in improving the public's health. The strategy also aims to ensure that patients, carers and the public have the information necessary to make decisions about their own treatment and care, and to influence the shape of health services generally.
>
> (National Health Service Executive 1998: 9)

Thus the resulting shape of the service emerging from this strategy deployment should be one characterised by its effective use of information resources, where flows of information and knowledge feed innovation and flexibility, and where great emphasis is placed upon putting the citizen or user at the centre of these processes.

It is worth exploring in greater detail the concepts outlined in the NHS strategy, in respect of the issues of good practice that they allude to, but also with regard to some of the key questions around exclusion where, it is possible to argue, many questions remain both unasked and unanswered. If we consider what is set out as the UK government's vision of a modern and appropriate health service, we learn among other things that it is viewed as critical that it should be:

- a national service;
- fast and convenient;
- of a uniformly high standard;
- designed around the needs of patients, not institutions;
- efficient, so that every pound is spent to maximise the care for patients;
- making good use of technology and know-how;
- tackling the causes of ill-health as well as treating it.

(National Health Service Executive 1998: 11)

Underpinning all of these statements of intent, it is possible to make linkages throughout the ambitious list to the part that IKM methodologies and approaches might play in delivering key objectives. However, one must also be cautious, taking note of the various 'health warnings' that have been signalled throughout this text, and consider whether some of these key points are in danger of being over-emphasised in respect of what they may actually contribute. Thus, an IKM strategist seeking to take the necessary holistic view of such strategy development, might ask how we ensure that, in seeking to be user-centric rather than organisationally focused, the technologies we deploy do not represent inflexible and barrier-creating structures in themselves. Likewise, how do we actually ensure that various levels of 'know-how', or knowledge, are fed into issues of prevention? The purpose of an overarching IKM strategy must therefore be, at least in part, to ask and seek to answer the questions of how full or even partial integration of policy objectives and targets can take place within a coherent framework.

Having said that, there are dangers around the issue of making rather too many assumptions that statements can be accepted as 'given'. What is particularly laudable in respect of the *Information for Health* strategy is that it does appear to have been underpinned by at least some sense of properly thought-through focus upon the role of information and, to a lesser extent, knowledge within the organisation as a whole. The scale and scope of such an undertaking should not be underestimated, nor the opportunities for learning from the way in which principles and objectives are set out. Importantly, though perhaps at times superficially, it could be argued that the strategy identifies the audience for its proposed changes as being comprised of four distinct yet mutually dependent groups: patients, health-care professionals; managers and planners; and the public (National Health Service Executive 1998: 16).

In respect of patients and their engagement with an IKM-focused health service, it is said:

> Patients and their carers are increasingly interested to learn more about their condition, the treatments they are undergoing, and the likely outcomes, as well as needing information to support them in day-to-day living with long-term conditions and in helping them access health and social care services.
>
> The prime source of such information will continue to be health-care professionals with whom they are in contact, but it is important that all the information they get – whether directly from those professionals or other sources – should be reliable.
>
> (National Health Service Executive 1998: 16)

If one were to ask a key question here with regard to the potential impact on addressing potential issues of exclusion, it would be around the extent to which there is a need for patients to be pro-active in their information-seeking behaviour. All of the issues previously discussed around possible identifiers of exclusion should leave one with a desire to seek answers to questions such as how you can ensure that information is supplied in appropriate patient-centred formats. Issues around access to other aspects of health and social services are likely, for many of the most excluded groups, to be the most critical linking information that they receive, but there must surely be a recognition that the information provided may need to be particularly tailored to ensure appropriateness to certain groups, and to some extent the degree of pro-activity may need to switch from an apparent emphasis upon the requirement for a 'curious' patient to strategies for ensuring information provision – and, through it, mechanisms for longer-term service delivery – for those who do not conform to an identified pattern of user behaviour.

When discussing the role of the health care professional within the information strategy, it is argued that they need:

> fast, reliable and accurate information about the individual patients in their care ... fast, easy access to local and national knowledge bases that support the direct care of patients and clinical decision making ... access to information to support them in the evaluation of the care they give.
>
> (National Health Service Executive 1998: 16)

Once more, this is an important articulation of the pivotal role that information resources and access to them can play in the delivery of key aspects of public service provision. However, it is also possible to question the extent to which this is articulated as primarily a passive process. The model presented here is one based upon the primacy of a one-way information delivery system and, of course, one cannot argue that this must be a critical part of delivering sound IKM practice. However, while there is clear reference to accessing knowledge bases and patient records, there is a singular lack of emphasis upon the importance of encouraging participation in the knowledge generation and sharing processes. This apparent omission, particularly when viewed within a context that is seeking to consider the role that IKM methodologies can play in positively impacting upon issues of social exclusion, must raise the question of how exactly it is envisaged that learning can take place and how observations, strategies and solutions deployed in a health care context can be shared. Where good practice is developed in ensuring, for example, systems for ensuring proper and effective linkage between a range of social services needed by an elderly, non-native-speaking citizen, IKM best practice would suggest that mechanisms for adding this to appropriate and accessible knowledge bases should be prioritised. The danger, as presented here, is that partial attempts at IKM will improve the service experience enjoyed by the majority of users, but will not achieve tangible impact upon those who, for a variety of reasons, do not conform to a common model of characteristics, behaviour, or both.

Much the same criticisms as those outlined above could be reasonably levelled at the discussion of information provision for policy-makers and managers, where there is, it is suggested, a clearly understood need:

> for managers and planners at every level in the service to have good quality information to help them to better target and use the resources deployed in the NHS and to improve the quality of life of patients and local communities.
>
> (National Health Service Executive 1998: 17)

Once more, there is little that one could disagree with in this statement. We know that good practice requires that the underpinning IM is the primacy of the requirement to have ready access to information resources in the right place, at the right time and in the right format. However, the question is again the degree of passivity that is suggested by the strategy document, and one would have to acknowledge that the aspiration of making a difference to both patients and to the wider local community would be likely to require something a good deal more interactive. Certainly, it is true to say that this strategy document, taken in isolation from the context of ongoing structural reform in the UK health service, does perhaps raise some issues regarding the gradual emergence of new modes of operation, with a more natural and seamless integration of service provision across traditional provider boundaries, and that these have not been fully taken into account in this discussion. However, this should not diminish the requirement in IKM terms, at a strategy level in particular, to clearly set out the need for pro-active and dynamic models of information sharing and knowledge exchange to be identified as priorities, at the very least, if they are to achieve real impact in the operational situation.

Turning to consider the role of 'the public' within the NHS information strategy, this is perhaps the most unsatisfactory area of discussion contained within the document, reflecting, at best, only partial understanding of the value of dynamic information and knowledge flows originating from the citizen as end-user; thus the impression given is of an essentially one-way process of information provision:

> The public wants the opportunity to access information such as good health and lifestyle advice. But people are also interested in understanding how the health service is performing in the delivery of health care services, both in terms of the efficiency of the service – for example, as indicated by waiting lists and waiting times – and also increasingly in its effectiveness in terms of outcomes.
>
> (National Health Service Executive 1998: 17)

Such a statement may certainly be true for a proportion of health service users, but it demonstrates no awareness of the possible importance of ensuring that some degree of *connectivity* with the end-user should take place. Here, the information flow is in a single direction: it flows down to the consumer, but does not acknowledge that it may be provided at a level and in formats which effectively serve to disenfranchise large swathes of citizens from accessing it and then making sense of it. Still more importantly, it omits all elements of the potential for driving forward organisational learning through ensuring that information and knowledge flows are capable of moving upwards as well as down.

The absence of emphasis upon building priorities into the information strategy to ensure opportunities for learning from the experience and perceptions of end-users as stakeholders, indicates a critical lack of awareness of what such a strategy should be capable of achieving. When considering the possible impact upon amelioration of certain aspects of social exclusion, it is possible, in an IKM context, to argue that the outcomes articulated within the NHS strategy, no matter how well meant, are likely simply to perpetuate patterns of exclusion. However, as we have also discussed in this chapter, formal consultation exercises with certain identified 'marginal groups' are likely to have little tangible impact upon the quality of input to planning processes. Thus, what we are left with may be a pattern of information management across a large and complex organisation which is contributing to, and in some circumstances actually validating, policy and subsequent service outcomes, and this in isolation from any consideration of those users who are not, for a variety of reasons, inputting to the information and knowledge sharing process. And if, as was suggested earlier in this chapter, a high proportion of service use actually emanates from the 'excluded' or non-involved user constituencies, how can it be legitimately argued that more efficient, effective and user-centred services will result?

Adding the missing IKM dimension to organisational information strategies

Although within the particular context of this book it is possible to posit the view that the information strategy produced by the UK NHS is flawed, it should be recognised that its very existence is an extremely positive move forward when considering public sector IKM applications. However, as with all new developments, there are dangers inherent in moving forward with a tool of organisational improvement which may actually serve to embed still further areas of practice which are at best limiting and, at worst, may be discriminatory. What may result is, of course, something less than service revolution, and rather more the mandating of internally held views around procedures and delivery mechanisms. It is important, too, to note that such a criticism should not be particularised to the health sector; rather, it should be seen as something that is generalisable across the spectrum of public service provision. The question therefore must be: how can an IKM focus serve to make organisations operate in a manner which demonstrates cognisance of the requirements of a diversity of stakeholding groups?

The key concept here must be the pivotal importance of building learning opportunities into any strategy. As Senge *et al.* discuss, a key determinant of success in harnessing the full value of IKM assets is the degree of integration and appropriate dissemination that can be achieved, drawing upon the diverse range of inputs that are both possible and desirable:

> Information that teams and individuals have generated cannot be fully understood in isolation from the rest of the system. ... The World Health Organization (WHO) learned the importance of this phase during the 1960s, during its world-wide campaign to eradicate smallpox. Experts assumed that the vaccination techniques which worked in the first locale, Tonga, could easily roll out to the entire planet. But in various countries, caseworkers needed a variety of strategies to work effectively with shortages, community attributes (some countries had extensive midwife networks), media (some countries had radio networks), and other local practices (like tattooing of nomadic water holes).
>
> All of their varied approaches were systematically recorded, and field workers received summary reports and supplemental papers every two to three weeks. Requests for help from the field got the highest priority responses at the central office. Staff people were expected to visit each country in their regions, at least once and preferably twice a year. Even embarrassing news, such as the politically sensitive locations of new outbreaks of the disease, was openly shared. Since everyone had access to all this information, WHO field workers continuously compared notes. ... This sharing of knowledge was critical to the ultimate success of the campaign.
>
> (Senge *et al.* 1999: 439)

What is most impressive in the World Health Organization example is that such foresight was deployed with regard to the prioritising of the dissemination of IKM resources and that it happened at a time when ICT applications were very much in their infancy. If we consider the tools we have available to us today that can be deployed to ensure that access to information across geographical and even organisational boundaries is facilitated, then it is legitimate ask why it is apparently such a neglected area. It is possible to argue that for most public sector organisations it may be because such a focus upon integrating and disseminating experience and observations is an alien concept. Globally, public sector structures are largely delineated by their emphasis upon procedures, protocols and hierarchies, and to introduce an element of learning and change, based upon tapping into information and knowledge resources held by a range of stakeholders, is a culturally difficult concept to 'sell'.

However, consideration of issues of social exclusion provides perhaps the most effective lobbying tool for addressing such neglect of opportunity. There is a discernible trend across the public sector to make access to public services more inclusive, and through this to minimise the degree to which citizens are marginalised within society. However, just as in the example of the World Health Organization it was quickly acknowledged that treating humanity as one homogeneous mass for the purposes of delivering a service was doomed at the outset to produce less than satisfactory outcomes, so too must public sector strategists acknowledge the dangers inherent in seeking to perpetuate models of service design and delivery that are informed by one-way and partial information flows.

Building mechanisms for sharing information and knowledge both within and between strata of public sector provision offers the single most important opportunity for working towards overcoming issues of citizen exclusion. Where the NHS information strategy is flawed, and many others follow the same pattern, is in the apparent assumption that, at the end-user level, the information flow is one-way, top-down: 'People need easy access to good quality information to enable them to influence local service development, as well as local and national policy' (National Health Service Executive 1998: 17).

Yet how many end-users are actually likely to engage in such levels of participation? And, are those who do choose to engage in this type of policy dialogue likely to be those who are already articulate and relatively demanding consumers of public services? The answers to these questions suggest that such a framing of strategy aspiration is likely to lead to the voices and concerns of relatively few being heard, and highlight the essentially limited impact that any such model might be capable of having on overcoming issues of exclusion.

Capitalising on IKM opportunities

Adoption of information and knowledge management strategies can undoubtedly lead to the development of more effective and efficient public sector organisations and, in a sense, if they contribute in this way then this should be viewed as a considerable achievement in itself. However, through the deployment of strategic foresight, it is possible to argue that the outcomes of IKM applications can be leveraged still further, through the recognition that they are capable of acting as major contributors to any political agenda that prioritises the minimisation of social exclusion.

Principles around information and knowledge sharing represent the key to identifying particular and appropriate strategies for providing services to, and engaging in dialogue with, individuals and communities who have been less than well served by traditional public sector structures. Acknowledging this means recognising that learning from experience and observation must be treated as a priority, and therefore requires the support of properly thought-through operational protocols to facilitate the levels of sharing and exchange that can actually make a difference to the experience of the end-user. Facilitating this might well involve identifying clusters of public sector activity, managed through different departments or agencies, but where there are clear synergies in respect of linkages that the citizen may experience at the point of use: for instance, benefits and employment services, health services and social care provision, and ensuring that good practice and observations can be recorded and subsequently accessed in a meaningful manner.

On the whole, the direct input of the most 'disadvantaged' members of society is unlikely to be readily forthcoming, and the likelihood is that real opportunities for learning and developing more tailor-made and successful services will be created by engaging front-line service employees in the process of thinking about the implications of the transactions they engage in as part of their daily routine of client contact, and providing a mechanism for them to share their ideas and views. Critically, for this to work it has to become embedded in the organisational culture and to be seen as something that is very much part of the responsibility of each employee, where benefits accruing from using shared information and knowledge are celebrated for the positive impact that they may have on service design and delivery mechanisms.

It is also important that, within an agenda of seeking to reduce instances of exclusion within society, public service structures must show themselves to be willing to engage 'third parties' in the learning and knowledge exchange process. Involving community and voluntary groups, which may have readier access to those who, for a variety of factors, are at a disadvantage in their dealings with public sector bodies, is an eminently sensible way forward. However, as with so much that has been discussed in relation to the impact which IKM is capable of bringing to public sector organisations, the greatest challenge is represented by the suggestion that something which undermines the traditional and departmentally insular operating structure should become the organisational operating norm.

Skewing the communications channels: illusory participation

Within the context of this discussion of issues around promoting the degree of inclusion within society generally, a key argument to note is that put forward by advocates of the democratising premise thought to emerge from increasing penetration of Internet access. Such a view will typically argue that society more generally will display a greater willingness to engage in debate around political and public service issues as more and more citizens become users of this tool, which of course primarily facilitates communication rather than simply being a channel of passive information. However, while it may be true to say that there is certainly a trend emerging which sees the Internet being used increasingly as a forum for lobbying, the expression of dissatisfaction and the engagement of many citizens in what might be termed 'pressure group' activities, this is most certainly not the case for those key groups of intensive public service users who are, for a variety of factors, often marginalised by society.

Thus, while it is clearly important to acknowledge that the Internet and the essentially unstructured and open flow of communication that it affords may be beneficial for many in society, giving them avenues for making their views known, it cannot be held that this necessarily means that the most critical issues of exclusion will necessarily benefit from this process. So while the input of citizens into a range of discussion and exchange fora on the Internet is undoubtedly going to provide a major source of ideas and views which can be usefully fed into public service reform, it will remain important to acknowledge that there are possibly some key 'voices' missing from this particular dialogue.

A vision of IKM benefits in the area of social exclusion

Contributing to the development of a model of society where far fewer citizens are marginalised and effectively excluded is potentially the area of greatest long-term benefit that IKM can deliver to public service. However, analysis of present practice would suggest that so far the full potential has not yet been released in any model of service strategy or plan. Therefore, a key challenge for the IKM strategist must be to build in, and make seamless, opportunities for the exchange and sharing of ideas and observations, be this internally, cross-departmentally or through effective 'hook up' with external third party agencies. Technologies can certainly help to facilitate this, with Intranets – and extranets in the case of third party co-operation – representing considerable opportunities. However, without a properly thought-through and coherent focus upon what is actually required and how potential contributors will be educated and persuaded regarding the value of participation in such a way, the likelihood is that, although models of public service delivery may change, levels of exclusion will remain virtually unchanged.

Chapter 9

Vision and revision
The case for IKM in the public sector

Establishing a credible and persuasive case for the adoption of IKM-based methodologies in the public sector represents a major challenge for those charged with leading forward reform and change into the twenty-first century. From the outset, it has been argued that to couch strategies for the adoption of an IKM focus in anything other than the language of improvement and value-adding activity is to invite the almost inevitable certainty of it being treated as a marginal and largely peripheral activity. However, as we have discussed in the preceding chapters, issues around the management of information and knowledge are absolutely central to the way in which public sector organisations operate, and they also hold the key for the achievement of many of the reform agendas currently discussed in major global economies. In this, our concluding section, it is important to consider the strategies that will see IKM practice becoming embedded in public sector practice. The very real barriers and difficulties that such an approach will face require not only *vision* on the part of those charged with leading efforts in this area, but also confidence and ability, linked with a clear mandate and the authority to effect *revisions*.

Providing IKM vision

To seek to provide organisational vision and associated structure to the areas of information and knowledge requires a level of understanding and thought leadership the like of which the public sector has rarely, to date, been able to call upon. To be a credible thought leader requires, as we discussed in the opening chapters of this text, considerable command of the specialist area, as well as the important skill of being able to communicate with and enthuse key constituent groups to achieve high levels of both understanding of and commitment to the IKM-driven change agenda. However, such an articulation of perceived organisational need requires that at least two deceptively straightforward questions are asked: how do you ensure that the role of the IKM leader is identified as being not only an organisational requirement but, most importantly, a senior-level one? And, if the need for such an appointment is recognised, where are you going to recruit your IKM leader from?

Questions such as these can operate at a number of levels, from the macro position of looking at policies and strategies for national governments through to responsibility for departmental or local service applications. However, in a sense it must be true to say that, unless there is the macro-level acknowledgement of the importance of IKM issues and a recognition that they require leadership and management, then no matter how good local initiatives may be, they can never fully achieve their potential. The view that IKM requires a climate and soil in which it can flourish, articulated from the outset, remains very much a requirement of the achievement of a vision that sees the public sector utilising and extracting value from its information and knowledge assets. Thus, the organisational environment is critical, and occasional rhetoric referring to the importance of the 'information society' or the 'knowledge economy' will never be enough to turn a neglected and overgrown area into a fertile and productive vista.

In IKM terms, having the vision to move from a position of neglect, although arising more from ignorance and misunderstanding of the worth and potential of the asset base than from any more deliberate position, is a task that must be tackled at many levels if successful outcomes are to be achieved. Both a strength and a potential weakness in moving this particular agenda forward is the fact that the terms *information* and *knowledge* have become so ubiquitous within the wider political lexicon. They are used widely by politicians and senior public sector managers, but they are too rarely referred to in ways that would, upon some closer analysis, stand up alongside the principles and methodologies outlined within the framework of this text. The question posed here is: how can issues of IKM, which represent potentially major changes to and re-evaluation of accepted public sector modes of working, effectively enter and impact upon the thought processes of those who are empowered to require and mandate new ways of working?

IKM vision and the role of the politician

The democratic principle of public governance sets out tremendous expectations of, and responsibilities for, those who hold high elected office. Theirs is a responsibility to provide both leadership and vision, a role for which, in some cases, they may be said to be unprepared. Public sector reform, as with almost any type of significant organisational change, is almost always a process that is driven from the higher echelons of power, and as such relies for the credibility of outcomes of policies and strategies upon the confidence and clarity of thought provided by those leading such activities. However, within this context, and reflecting once more upon the complexity and often intangible nature of information and knowledge assets, we must surely ask how elected politicians can reach a position of championing issues of IKM.

The difficulties facing elected politicians are persuasively outlined by Goddard and Riback who, taking the United States as their case study of a mature democracy, expose both the strengths and the weaknesses of moving forward truly innovative and informed change agendas within an elected system of governance:

> Our democracy was designed to allow people from all walks of life the chance to serve a stint in public office ... This turnover of government officials brings vitality and freshness. Few Americans want a permanent government. But there is, of course, a downside. Lots of it. Though we elect and appoint officials to government who have little relevant experi- ence – Robert Reich went from managing half the time of one secretary to more than 18,000 employees and a $35 billion dollar budget when he moved from Harvard professor to U.S. Labor Secretary – we expect government to run well. With Capitol Hill offices facing turnover every two years, this 'government of novices' is a perpetual problem.
>
> (Goddard and Riback 1998b: 1)

In itself, such a scenario is worrying, for we have articulated here a view of elected politicians as providing a necessary dynamic for moving forward the development of an IKM culture within the public sector, yet it would seem that few of them are actually in a position to take on this key role as political champion for IKM reform. However, this is perhaps to underesti- mate the importance of the organisational 'novice'. New entrants to the halls of political power are in a uniquely privileged position to be able to ask questions of the structure and operation of the organisational model that delivers their policies and strategies. Those entering the political arena with recent experience of organisational practice in other sectors should be well placed to ask questions around approaches to the management of informa- tion and knowledge assets and, on the basis of this, to contribute to the evolution of a serious and questioning view of what the public sector is doing to promote the maximisation of the value of these assets. Only a minority will be in a position to do this credibly, but it is through this asking of questions by politicians, a querying of accepted and established modes of operation, that the role of the political novice is potentially of central importance in moving forward the public sector IKM agenda.

Key pointers to ways in which politicians should take control of their role and responsibilities are provided by Goddard and Riback, who have identi- fied what they refer to as *The Eight Traits of Highly Successful Public Officials*, detailing how politicians have a responsibility for taking charge of and giving direction to their organisational and societal role in government (Goddard and Riback 1998a). In relation to issues of IKM, it is helpful to focus upon three of the traits identified, for they serve to give considerable weight and direction to the potential role of the politician in driving forward an IKM agenda.

In the first instance, they argue that politicians operating at an appropriate level of seniority should 'rethink government's main purpose':

> Many new public officials find themselves heading agencies where the day-to-day work goes beyond what they expected. With management teams swept in and out over the years, most agencies perform tasks they should not. Some government functions are more appropriate for the private sector, some overlap with other agencies and some are simply no longer relevant.
>
> (Goddard and Riback 1998a: 2)

However, the achievement of such a reconceptualisation and rationalisation of what is meant by, and delivered by, the public sector is in effect an IKM-intensive exercise. All of the issues around information and associated workflow, driving forward learning based upon tapping into knowledge networks and reducing overall levels of duplication and waste alluded to here, flow back inevitably to the achievement of key principles of IKM. If senior-level politicians accept that they have a critical responsibility for at least inputting into the rethinking of the role and structure of public services, then there must surely be an allied emphasis upon adopting the very tools which are going to deliver properly constructed change in these areas.

Goddard and Riback further argue that a key attribute of the successful politician must be some sense that they 'know what they want to accomplish':

> Little could sound more obvious. After all, who would run for office or accept appointment to an important government position without having a clear idea of what to achieve or how government should perform? Yet stop a random congressman in the halls of the Capitol and too often you'll find they lack what President George Bush called 'the vision thing.'
>
> (Goddard and Riback 1998a: 2)

Taking a lead on issues around an IKM-driven public sector represents a challenge and an opportunity for those politicians who can demonstrate a clear grasp of the reform agenda represented. A vision of 'better government' or 'modern government' will only be effective if underpinned by some clarity of exactly what it is that must be accomplished to make the laudable but intrinsically rather abstract vision a reality. An ability to deliver on the vision is a key requirement of those who aspire to the highest levels of political leadership; as such, the potential held out by the adoption of IKM principles should provide much which is attractive to those with both personal and political ambition for advancement, simply because the potential outcomes in respect of service enhancement and efficiency gains are so very great.

The third of the traits or recommendations made to politicians is the often daunting challenge of taking control of the bureaucracy which surrounds them in office:

> Empowering bureaucrats is today's conventional wisdom in making government work. It is also wrong. Instead top new public officials must learn to empower themselves. They must liberate themselves from the multiple layers of bureaucracy and arcane rules that block their ability to take control of their agency. The permanent bureaucracy, originally designed to prevent abuse, now insulates public officials from the people so that empowering bureaucrats actually decreases government's accountability.
>
> (Goddard and Riback 1998a: 3)

Freeing up the process of change in the public sector remains, despite almost two decades of reform, a live issue for politicians who wish to challenge embedded practices and perceptions of roles and responsibilities. Putting in place an IKM-driven change agenda is likely, at some levels at least, to represent a profoundly uncomfortable and perhaps even threatening proposition for significant numbers of public sector employees. Linking to the need for political vision and the drive to see this translated into action, a key challenge for the politician who leads on an IKM-focused change agenda must be the ability and determination to persuade those who remain sceptical and resistant to change, and it may be that this group will include not only a proportion of employees but also, almost certainly, a number of fellow politicians who do not share the same vision of public sector improvement mediated by greater focus upon the role and value of information and knowledge assets.

Delivering on the vision: the role of the IKM leader

The requirement that politicians take a lead on, and provide ongoing commitment to, the achievement of an IKM-focused change agenda has been clearly stated. However, what remains a critical issue is who, at a senior level, is going to take forward key issues of transforming policy statements into strategies which are capable of being successfully operationalised.

Within a competent and highly professional public sector career structure, there is as yet little evidence that the role of the IKM leader and manager has been recognised and defined with any degree of clarity. Yet if we contrast this with employment trends emerging in other sectors, particularly in service industries, we can begin to see a clear demand for senior-level managers in the IKM area, commanding premium salary packages, becoming apparent in recruitment activity. Against this background of shortage of the core skills at an appropriate level, and the need for start-up expertise to be fed into public sector strategy development, it may be that the only option for the public sector in the short term is to seek to recruit IKM leaders externally, or to buy in consultancy expertise in this area. Both such options of course, are often intrinsically problematic to enact successfully.

Let us consider the first potential option for public sector operations: that they should seek to recruit expertise in IKM from another sector. This is not, of course, an unusual proposition, with much reform of the last twenty years having been underpinned by a view that recruiting from the commercial sector can help to sharpen the focus of public services. However, a number of questions emerge if we explore this option, the first and most important being: at what level are you going to 'import' your IKM leader? By this what is meant is that IKM principles and practices represent such a new undertaking for a majority of public sector organisations, and such a key challenge to the traditional functional structures of public services, that, in the first instance at least, making appointments to individual departments may actually have limited benefit in the achievement of IKM gains across and between various operating strands of government. Thus, a critical first stage may be to identify where IKM leaders may be located, in order that they can be in a position to assess and develop strategies for improvements across the whole of public service operations. The key role here, then, becomes one of giving policy guidance to politicians and enacting the development of strategies which are capable of rolling out across diverse and often apparently unconnected strands and tiers of public service.

It should be immediately apparent that the role outlined above is a considerable one, where influencing and communication skills, as well as possession of a considerable grasp of IKM theory, would be key requirements. Whether it is desirable that such a role should be filled by an established IKM leader from another sector is open to question. Certainly, as has been said in support of the role of politicians, it is undoubtedly important that there are people who see one of their key responsibilities to be that of challenging the *status quo*. An external appointment is therefore certainly an opportunity in this respect, whereby longstanding assumptions around structures, practices and the characteristics of the operating culture can be questioned on the basis of the IKM leader being at some remove from them and possibly bringing experience of other operating cultures. However, there are also considerable dangers inherent in recruiting your IKM leader externally, and these are primarily framed in terms of the potential lack of understanding of the complexity, unique mission and operating position which defines, even today, much of what we understand by the public sector. It may be that an external appointment in this key area actually invites early failure rather than the quick wins so desirable in driving forward the adoption and embedding of IKM strategies.

Adopting the practice of buying in consultancy expertise to provide first-level leadership for IKM effort is certainly a possibility, and one for which major global management consultancies are undoubtedly readying themselves. However, as with the argument around making a very senior-level external appointment, caution must be shown around letting contracts with external companies on the basis that IKM 'solutions' may be provided. The offer of a 'solution' in respect of IKM should, in itself, ring many alarm bells, for it is not a 'quick fix' approach to reengineering your organisation: rather, it must be viewed as something much more organically based, the benefits of which emerge over time. Similarly, when requiring an external consultancy to develop strategies for IKM implementation, the scope of the undertaking must be questioned: would they, for example, be providing macro-level recommendations that would flow out through the various tiers of government, or would they be required to take a much more functionally based, strand-by-strand approach to their work?

In essence, there is no easy answer to the questions posed here, either around the suitability of making a senior-level external appointment and/or employing external consultants to deliver high-level strategic direction. If there is significant political sign-up to the principles of IKM-enabled public sector reform then this has to be actioned in some way, but the key question remains: how? Delivering on a political vision of IKM will require leadership, and it is certainly true to say that the type and level of leadership needed, in terms of the characteristics and actual numbers of people employed, will vary depending upon the scale of ambition associated with the reform agenda.

A possible model of good practice for nation-states would require that there was considerable political commitment to the vision of transforming public sector use of information and knowledge assets. From this emerges an obvious need: that within government, at the highest level, IKM should be led and managed with a degree of visibility and authority commensurate with its importance, possibly even alongside the revenue or treasury function. To operate successfully at this level, there has to be a clearly articulated clarity of vision and underpinning authority, which positions the IKM leader at the centre of public sector operations.

From a central position within government, IKM is then mandated to feed out of and into various functions and strata of public sector operation. Moving to such a position represents a radical repositioning of the role and importance of IKM within the public sector, and would not necessarily be achieved without some considerable resistance from key opinion leaders operating at senior levels across public service operations. The challenge of overcoming scepticism and resistance to change, particularly at an early stage, where the resistors are likely to be other senior-level managers, is perhaps one of the main reasons why high-level and sustained commitment from politicians is a key requirement for IKM success, but is also a factor which mitigates against external consultants being the channel to deliver first-level IKM leadership. To hand over responsibility for making an early stage case for activity in this area, and in a sense providing a *de facto* thought leadership role, is to invite accusations of a credibility gap in the approach to IKM being promoted. For if, after all, IKM is about utilising assets that are primarily internally generated and held in a different and more effective way, then responsibility for moving forward on this basis must also be seen to be held internally.

Thus, where at all possible, it would seem sensible that the IKM reform leader should be appointed on the basis of having had some senior-level experience of working within the public sector. In drawing up an appropriate person specification, emphasis should be placed upon traits including demonstrable success as a leader of major projects and as a gifted communicator and negotiator, ideally with some experience of IKM initiatives. It might well be that those making such a senior-level appointment will wish to utilise opportunities for looking outside discrete national boundaries for the best candidates to fulfil this specification; indeed, for many countries the likelihood is that such people simply do not exist within their operating structures. Thus, the reality of supply and demand in the area of senior-level IKM appointments may mean that, as these positions emerge, some degree of head-hunting of suitable candidates will result, possibly with the benefit of making the flow of public sector personnel across national boundaries more of a reality than at present.

However, as has been stated, the pool of candidates for such senior-level positions is extremely small, and the likelihood is that compromise appointments will result, some of which may be based upon recruitment from other sectors with a likelihood that much early-stage IKM policy and strategy development work will be carried out by external consultancies. Such a position does not, of course, mean that failure is inevitable; rather, there are perhaps even more factors which need to be taken into account when setting out on a journey designed to transform political vision into applied reality. One key factor in achieving long-term benefits is that the public sector must invest in developing its own IKM expertise at senior, middle and operational levels and in identifying this area particularly as a career strand and opportunity for the most able and ambitious recruits into the public sector.

Undoubtedly, delivering on the vision with regard to IKM is going to be almost totally reliant upon the quality of the people charged with leading and operationalising activities in this area. There are considerable dangers inherent in adopting the structures and approaches discussed, but they are as nothing if the wrong people are appointed in the first instance to key

IKM positions. Where these people are going to be recruited from is certainly a major and currently extremely live issue, for the pool of available talent is very small. However, assuming that short-term issues around leadership can be overcome, an opportunity for developing a new generation of public sector managers who are comfortable with and capable in aspects of IKM must be addressed with some urgency.

Further, embedding IKM principles in public sector organisational cultures is essentially a proposition that is predicated upon the achievement of appropriate levels of education, training and communication, to ensure that the vision is shared and enacted. Such a position cannot be achieved without much foresight, substantial resourcing and considerable commitment from political leaders, who are informed and advised by their most senior-level IKM managers. The key principle here is the potential revolution represented by moving towards the widespread adoption of IKM-driven principles of operation; these have to be treated as evolutionary concepts, and as such, the costs and benefits – and indeed the planning processes to support such activities, particularly in ensuring that there is an emerging IKM-literate workforce – must be viewed over a period of some years rather than according to the often short-termist perspective which has too often dominated critical aspects of public sector reform.

Developing a new public sector culture

Time and senior-level commitment would, therefore, appear to be the two crucial ingredients in moving to a credible position of IKM-focused public sector management, and it is by no means certain that these inputs will always, or indeed often, be made available. However, at the commencement of the twenty-first century there is at least an acknowledgement by politicians that society is evolving in ways that are impacted upon and in some cases mediated by the continuing emergence of the pivotal role of information and knowledge assets. Such a recognition is at least helpful in moving many of the issues raised within this text to a more prominent role. However, one simple fact remains: IKM benefits cannot be simply parachuted into the public sector. Rather, they will have to be built over time and become the underpinning architecture of a new public sector operating culture.

If it is to deliver the benefits of IKM alluded to, the culture referred to must be focused upon people – people as employees and people as citizens. It must consider the enabling role that technology can play in bringing public services into alignment with the way in which the majority of populations live their lives today, rather than shackling them to structures and modes of delivery informed by outdated practices. That this is 'revolutionary' is to overstate the case, for the public sector globally has shown itself capable of being reformed, although the changes instigated have usually been compartmentalised and focused upon maintaining or merely 'tweaking' the stovepipe applications and structures which are the legacy of the Victorian era.

In this book we have considered a number of examples of the reform agenda being enacted in Australia, where important questions have been asked and solutions posited around the creation of a mode of public service appropriate for a modern nation-state. It is important to critically review what is happening in this context, from the creation of a national policy on information management through to the ambitious plans for Centrelink services and the more local take-up of these directions, such as the innovative approaches adopted by Brisbane City Council. What this emphasises is the importance and impact of having clear direction at the macro level, and the likelihood that this will have consequences that radiate out through all tiers of public sector delivery. Thus, a political lead has been set at a senior national policy level; this has been acted upon through the reengineering of services provided by central government, and this in turn has given a clear lead to other strata of government as to the way in which they should be seeking to move forward their own change agenda. Fundamentally, the parameters for the culture and climate of public services have been set, and some five years into the change agenda we have had the opportunity to consider the way in which these are becoming embedded and operationalised.

Creating such cultures and climates, ready and able to enact significant change, is possibly the greatest challenge that the public sector faces today. A key difficulty is the lack of understanding among politicians of the limitations that technologies have in enacting change. Indeed, one has only to read newspaper accounts of chaos arising from the transfer to an ICT-mediated operating environment of services such as passport issuing and benefits payments to realise that it is naive in the extreme to expect technology alone to deliver new and improved models of public service provision. Successful change can only, in the end, result from thinking through what it is that you are managing and what you want to do with it, culminating in a position where you understand both your resources and your customers.

A major difficulty in the public sector, especially in the last two decades, which have seen reform agenda move firmly centre-stage, is that change implications have not been sufficiently well thought through; instead of a culture evolving which is receptive and flexible to change, one too often finds a demotivated and demoralised workplace environment and a citizen interface that is not engaged with the reform agenda. Thus, it is hardly surprising that very real barriers have been created to the achievement of an IKM-focused public sector; for example, widespread employee suspicion has become embedded as a core identifier of public sector culture, and this cannot simply be overcome through political rhetoric.

Thus, in addition to the 'vision thing' alluded to earlier in this chapter, there must be a clear acknowledgement at the most senior levels that the achievement of different ways of public sector working will require considerable recognition to be given to the need to take a longer-term view of achieving improvement. Taking down barriers between different operational areas of public service provision is something which, in reality, could be achieved overnight if there was political will to do so, but breaking down these barriers and achieving a culture where employees recognise the value and benefits of sharing information and knowledge with one another is an entirely different proposition. Legislating for new public sector structures may, in many instances, be a necessary statutory requirement, but it is only ever likely to be a cosmetic exercise if there is not considerable commitment and leadership given to actually making the changes work.

Realistically, political statements and legislation around public sector structures and delivery modes must be treated as a starting point on the road to 'better government', rather than being perceived as the culmination of the change process. Communicating with and gaining the sign-up of employees is the only sure way of moving forward, and for this to happen there must be a culture of openness and trust that is genuinely focused upon building and developing better ways of working. When such a culture evolves – and sadly there are as yet too few examples of such an environment being created – then there is every chance that the final contributor to the emergence of a truly IKM-enabled organisation, the service end-user, will become far more readily engaged in driving forward service development.

If IKM represents anything in terms of organisational culture, it is the need for engagement and openness to be championed. Suspicion, low morale and fear for longer-term employment security create a climate in which innovation is stifled and change resisted, a scenario which is all too familiar when taking a global overview of reform agenda in the public sector enacted since the early 1980s. A central premise of this text has been the primacy of information and knowledge assets in the public sector and their woeful neglect as something that might usefully be harnessed to drive forward new and more appropriate modes of working. Yet, if we are to believe much of the political rhetoric which has been prevalent at the close of the twentieth century, we are entering a period where the primacy of information and knowledge will be recognised and harnessed as never before. This sets up a major paradox, for we have, on the one hand, public sector cultures which are totally inappropriate for driving forward IKM-enabled change, and on the other, a political agenda which is informed at least by liberal reference to the primacy of information and knowledge as key drivers of change.

There are no easy answers to this apparent paradox. The model set out in this text demonstrates clearly that there are both barriers and opportunities associated with public sector adoption of IKM principles. However, critical success factors and the assignment of reasons for failure will almost always find their source as being in the way in which an organisation's people can engage with the challenges and changes presented to them. Short-termism is the key critical differentiator between the drivers of the public sector and the commercial sector; for the former, priorities are set by time-scales for re-election, whereas the latter can, and indeed should be expected to, take a view of the medium- and longer-term business opportunities. Changing public sector cultures means engaging politicians in a recognition that they must demonstrate a willingness to plan for a future which lies beyond the date of their next election, something which very few have shown themselves prepared to do. For IKM principles to become embedded and to flourish, there is, at the heart of the challenge presented by public sector applications, a need for acknowledgement that the process is owned not simply by politicians, but by all of those involved in the service delivery dynamic, from the most senior managers to the front-line staff and, through them, to the feeding in of the end-user perceptions and experiences of engagement with all tiers of public service.

Thus, an IKM organisational culture must be inclusive. Further, it must have the capacity to evolve over time. For these reasons alone there is a need for some considerable caution around discussions of potential benefits which may accrue to the public sector through the adoption of IKM practices. We have only to look at the way in which the public sector is littered with the apparent failures of improvement tools and techniques such as Business Process Reengineering (BPR) and Enterprise Resource Planning (ERP), often used successfully in the commercial sector, to question whether IKM might not suffer exactly the same fate. Reasons given for apparent non-returns upon investment made are couched in the all-too-familiar terminology of 'but we are different'. However, instead of focusing upon excuses that assert the primacy of 'difference', perhaps it is more accurate to suggest that failure accrues rather from poor application and insufficient time being assigned to the achievement of positive pay-backs before a new mode of working or organisational approach is prematurely assigned to the bulging public sector 'dustbin'. A controversial view, perhaps, but one which certainly bears thinking about when considering the pivotal importance of building an IKM-supporting public sector culture.

2020 vision: what will IKM-driven public services look like?

Throughout history, there has been a tradition that mankind constantly casts an eye to the future and envisages scenarios of what the world might conceivably look like. In this case, it is a useful exercise to cast one's eyes to the blue skies of the future and to consider what the public sector structures of the future will look like. How will citizens engage with them? How seismic is the scale and rate of change likely to be? The short answer is, of course, that we don't know, with any degree of certainty. However, looking at the trends emerging at the outset of the twenty-first century, it is possible to construct a view which suggests that things may be at once very different and still very much the same, at least in respect of key issues which need to be addressed on an ongoing basis.

What is likely to be very different, in democratic societies at least, is that drifts in levels of citizen participation will have been addressed in a range of ways. Perhaps the most likely is that, even in societies which have long held it to be an infringement of civil liberties, the requirement that citizens take part in political elections will have moved to a position whereby certain levels of participation in the democratic process are mandatory. Of course, supporting this may be the fact that for a majority of citizens participation will have become a great deal easier. Moves towards rolling out the use of electronic voting will have become embedded, and as this takes place and the technology becomes more and more familiar, it is possible to envisage a future scenario which will see opportunities for participation and comment on local, national and possibly even transnational issues being opened up on a far more regular basis.

The year 2020 will also see many of the most industrially developed countries in the world seeking to manage the problem of an increasingly ageing population and having to design and deliver a range of services which are appropriate for this significant sector of users. The promises held out by the 'information society' and the 'knowledge economy' will have found themselves particularly tested in respect of how the public sector has been able to develop appropriately to meet the needs and expectations of this sector of society. A generation who grew up with the promise of a technology-enabled 'better world' may conceivably find themselves in their 'third age', as post-retirement is sometimes euphemistically called, questioning how public sector structures are supporting their aspirations for improved quality of life.

In nations which are currently in a transitional stage into developed economies, huge changes in infrastructure are likely to result in considerable transformation of the ways in which people and communities relate to one another. Above all, the two-thirds of the world's population who currently do not have access to telephone-based communications are likely to see tremendous changes enacted through the increased penetration of this most basic of ICT tools. This will undoubtedly feed into the emergence of far greater focus upon the roles and responsibilities of public service providers, with many emerging economies being well placed to establish structures and approaches to service delivery unhindered by the (often) centuries of tradition evident in many more developed nations. So, it is possible to take a view that innovation and reform in the public sector will be global in scope, and that emerging economies may be able to enact IKM principles with considerably less emphasis upon the need to overcome barriers than will be the case for nations such as those considered as case studies in this text.

Perhaps the greatest change evident in the way that public services will look from a perspective of twenty years hence is that there is likely to be a much more logical and end-user focused approach to the way in which organisations operate. The current model, which typically sees a split of provision and responsibility across national, regional and sometimes local boundaries, is going to be challenged, possibly to the point of extinction. The questions that an IKM-focused reform agenda specifically asks, around the use of resources to best effect and the minimising of waste and duplication, will have resulted in the collapsing of many of the present artificial boundaries of provision. The first two decades of the twenty-first century could see real progress being made in marrying the goal of citizen-centric service provision with the aspiration to reduce the muddle and mess resulted in by lack of co-ordination across traditional stovepipe structures and applications.

By 2020, having responded to the challenges introduced by moving towards the maximisation of IKM assets, politicians and senior managers alike will be working within a structure which is capable of being more *personal*, inasmuch as the individual citizen should be enjoying the benefits to meaningful single entry points to public services, and at the same time more consensual and *participative*. Citizens, as end-users, will provide key and ongoing contributions to the development of services, with a culturally embedded mode of contributing to ongoing service development.

So there is every likelihood, if we take a view that IKM principles have been embraced and become embedded over time, that something which could genuinely be described as 'joined-up' public services could be realistically expected to result. These services will make use of increasingly powerful and sophisticated ICT applications, and as a result a majority of citizens and of the public service work force are likely to be operating in distinctly different ways from those which we observe today: the culture of both use and delivery should have moved on significantly. The concepts of space and time as key defining factors in relation to the availability of access to public services will have been largely eradicated. For a large majority of both questions and transactions, the citizen will be able to engage in communication with relevant services at locations and at times which are more convenient to them. Where public services continue to have a direct public access presence, it is likely that staff and facilities will be located within public spaces such as shopping centres, leisure complexes or health care facilities and that those staff at the front line will be generalists, capable of handling a full range of service queries and making linkages, possibly via video connection, to experts at remote locations. Such service points are also likely to be capable of addressing issues that cover all tiers of public service provision, with a complete removal, from public view at least, of a sense of separateness around different strata of government.

Thus, if looking to the future reveals a dominance of one key theme, it is surely that of increased momentum in tearing down many of the barriers and boundaries that operate across traditional models of public service provision. An interesting example of this crystal-ball gazing exercise was undertaken in 1998 by Cross, who, taking as his area of study the health sector and looking only as far forward as 2010, framed a number of interesting scenarios for what health care might look like. He considered first what an IKM-focused approach to ICT spend might achieve:

> Telemedicine can replace the need for a patient to move physically up the classic pyramid of care, from GP to district hospital to specialist academic centre. It will cut costs by reducing the number of inappropriate consultations. Maybe 40 per cent of patients could be referred by telemedicine.
>
> Electronic medical records will be available seamlessly to any authorised person who needs them. Knowledge filters will be able to recognise which particular types of clinician are trying to access the record. Suppose somebody has carotid artery disease and is referred to hospital for an ultrasound scan. The cardiologist reads the scan in his own specialist terms, not spelling out in detail all his conclusions. When, after discharge, the record gets back to the GP, the computer would apply this knowledge filter, decide that the GP needs more info and thus furnish some explanatory notes, or even an image – maybe a cartoon explaining exactly what's wrong in terms of the arterial plaque.
>
> Given access control, we can build a shared health record available to people who need it throughout the whole primary care team – including practice nurses, midwives, district nurses, health visitors. It may well include telemedicine. It certainly includes intelligent use of telephone technology, perhaps voice telephony and conferencing. Maybe others such as social services would have access to some part of the health record, though that is still controversial … Then you avoid all the duplication, and time wasted.
>
> (Cross 1998: 69–70)

Of course, health care represents a very distinct sector of public service and the scale and scope of changes envisaged here can have particular resonance for almost everyone. However, the underpinning message of IKM-driven change in the coming decades is generalisable, and it will be dominated by the emergence of far greater levels of coherence across functions in ways which will qualitatively improve the end-user experience of public service interaction. But what will it actually feel like to work within these new, more fluid structures? Indeed, how many people will still be able to define their employment status as 'public sector'? This last question is an important one if we are looking to the future, for the emergence of an IKM-facilitated mode of working does raise some important questions around the extent to which monopoly provider status will be preserved in the longer term for many of those core functions currently performed through directly managed departments and agencies. The emergence of operating cultures in the coming two decades, where sharing and cross-boundary working are enabled, may well result in far fewer directly employed public service workers, with many functions, such as call centre handling, being placed in the hands of contractors working to clearly defined parameters and with a strong emphasis upon the setting of both legal and operational limits to ensure that the public sector, as a whole, continues to benefit from the opportunities afforded by information and knowledge sharing.

Many of those remaining as employees of the public sector are likely to be working at higher-level policy and strategy positions, perhaps most often structured as cross-functional thematic groups, seeking to drive a continuously evolving change and improvement agenda forward across the whole of the public sector. It is possible that, as the nature and scope of such posts begin to emerge, public sector careers will once more become an attractive proposition, capable of attracting some of the most capable and innovative people in society to at least consider the public sector as a career option. Of course, as the nature of the public sector will have changed, so too will many of the ways in which individuals are employed, with possibly a majority of senior positions being moved from permanent contracts to rolling, performance-driven packages.

However, despite many of the very positive changes that it is possible to envisage IKM-driven developments delivering over the next two decades, there is also likely to be a very significant downside to the developments discussed above. As was discussed in some detail in Chapter 8, there is, at the commencement of the twenty-first century, a very real sense that issues of exclusion from society are becoming ever more problematic for very significant numbers of citizens. Developments in the IKM area, particularly around developing far better and more robust links to voluntary and community groups who may have easier access to certain of the most excluded groups in society, have been posited as a possible way of moving to address these critical issues. However, as models of public service delivery become more and more sophisticated, modelled on the needs and expectations of a majority of society, it is possible that we might well reach the year 2020 with exclusion being as real an issue then as it is for us today. Much, of course, will depend upon the determination and direction of politicians setting and driving forward the political agenda in the coming decades so that progress towards more inclusive models of society will actually be achieved. This remains perhaps the greatest question mark over the ultimate achievements that may be attributed to an IKM-driven reform programme: will it have a significant impact upon those who are perhaps most in need of public service support and guidance?

Courage and revision: the real critical success factors in public sector IKM

That much of this text has been about *potential* is undoubtedly true, for there are as yet very few really good examples of IKM practice visible within the public sector. But the direction and principles which might lead to significant and successful reform have been clearly stated; what is so far largely lacking is high-level informed commitment to delivering IKM-mediated public services. Certainly, as has been reflected upon, there is no shortage of rhetoric emerging from the mouths of politicians, or indeed embedded in policy documents, and yet analysis of the strategic and operational position of public sector provision across a number of continents provides evidence of only pockets of activity. There can thus be said to be something of a credibility gap: the theory of IKM is seized upon because it can usefully input into political sound bites, yet there is little evidence of top-level commitment to taking the opportunities offered to make a real difference to the way in which we all experience dealings with public sector operations.

If two ingredients are missing from the 'recipe' for the successful moving forward of IKM principles and practices, they can be said to be the unwillingness or absence of real courage on the part of senior politicians and public sector employees to rethink the way that the public service works, and from this base, a preparedness to revise and change as modes of service delivery evolve over time. The absence of the quality of courage to drive forward an IKM vision may certainly be attributed to political caution; less charitably, it may perhaps also be assigned to poor understanding of what is actually meant by taking control of public sector IKM assets. For far too many politicians, and indeed senior public sector managers, there remains a view that simply by sanctioning large-scale investment in ICTs, better public services will result. And yet, why should they? If your public services are found to be operating in a disjointed and fragmented manner, imposing a new and costly ICT architecture is not going to provide a miraculous transformation into a more rational and effective mode of working. Indeed, Caldow argues that the greatest dangers accruing from political focus on the benefits of the information society and the knowledge economy can be defined through what she refers to as the 'knowledge gap': put simply, politicians are happy to exhort the benefits of information and knowledge to public service reform, but probe beneath the surface and you will have difficulty in finding any real plans or strategies to bring about change (Caldow 1996: 24).

Politicians and senior-level managers will have to meet the challenge of closing the knowledge gap alluded to above if they are to make any gains in rethinking what it means to utilise information and knowledge assets within the public sector. Perhaps the most difficult issue facing this group is the extent to which rethinking needs to take place. This involves a concept increasingly referred to as 'imagineering': that is, displaying a willingness to conceive of structures and modes of delivery which are 'perfect', and to work towards their attainment, even if they may look radically different to the way in which services are currently delivered. However, what such an approach depends upon, and critically what also underpins the achievement of IKM-led improvements, is a willingness to acknowledge that the public sector needs to be prepared to abandon a mind-set where it accepts the literal 'price' of everything but recognises the 'value' of very little. And nowhere is this more true than in the way in which people and assets are regarded: for taking as a starting point a position that sees everything as a cost, rather than a potential contributor to improvement, will ultimately restrict innovation and enhance a culture where revision and change are often seen to result from failure, rather than from opportunities for learning and improvement. To move to this position, to realise the full potential of IKM in the public sector, will be almost entirely dependent upon the *vision*, *courage* and willingness to learn, as demonstrated by a preparedness to undertake service *revision*, that is evident among the most senior politicians and public service managers working today. The challenge of transforming *dinosaurs* into *dolphins*, introduced at the outset of this text, remains the key challenge and the key opportunity for moving to an IKM-mediated mode of service design and delivery.

Bibliography

Abell, A. (1994) 'Information uses and business success: a review of recent research in effective information delivery', in M. Feeney and M. Greeves (eds) *The Value and Impact of Information*, London: Bowker Saur.

Angel, I. (1998) 'The knowledge scam', *Information Strategy* 3, 6: 23–4.

Anthes, G. (1991) 'A step beyond a database', *Computerworld* 25, 9: 28.

Auster, E. and Choo, W. (1996) *Managing Information for the Competitive Edge*, New York: Neal-Schumann.

Australia, Information Management Steering Committee on Information Management in the Commonwealth Government (1997) *Management of Government Information as a National Strategic Resource*, Canberra, Australia: Office of Government Information Technology.

Bailey, R. (1997) 'Information: the currency of the new millennium', *International Information and Library Review* 29, 1: 36–42.

Baligh, H. (1994) 'Components of culture, nature, interconnections and relevance to decisions on organization structure', *Journal of Management Science* 40, 1: 14–27.

Battaglia, G. (1991) 'Strategic information planning: a corporate necessity', *Journal of Systems Management* February: 23–6.

Beer, M. (1990) 'Why change programs don't produce change', *Harvard Business Review* November–December: 158–66.

Benjamin, R. and Blunt, J. (1992) 'Critical IT issues: the next 10 years', *Sloan Management Review* Summer: 7–19.

Bensaou, M. and Earl, M. (1998) 'The right mind-set for managing information technology', *Harvard Business Review* September–October: 119–28.

Bird, J. (1996) 'It's all IT to me!', *Management Today* June, 78–81.

Blanton, J. (1992) 'Toward a better understanding of information technology organizations: a comparative case study', *MIS Quarterly* December: 531–55.

Boynton, A. (1993) 'Achieving dynamic stability through information technology', *California Management Review* Winter: 58–77.

Boynton, A. and Allen, B. (1991) 'Information architecture in search of efficient flexibility', *MIS Quarterly* December: 435–45.

British Productivity Council (1957) *Suggestion Schemes*, London: British Productivity Council.

Broadbent, M. and Samson, D. (1990) 'Improving the alignment of business and information strategies', unpublished working paper, University of Melbourne Graduate School of Management.

Brockman, J. (ed.) (1997) *Quality Management and Benchmarking in the Information Sector*, London: Bowker Saur.

Brooking, A. and Motta, E. (1996) 'A taxonomy of intellectual capital and a methodology for auditing it', unpublished proceedings of the seventeenth National Business Conference, Hamilton, Ontario, Canada, 24–6 January 1996.

Buchanan, S. and Gibb, F. (1998) 'The information audit: an integrated approach', *International Journal of Information Management* 18, 1: 29–47.

Burk, C. and Horton, F. (1988) *Infomap: A Complete Guide to Discovering Corporate Information Resources*, New York: Prentice Hall.

Burkitt-Gray, A. (1996) 'Something for everyone', *Electronic Government International* 1, 2: 14–15.

Burkitt-Gray, A. (1999) 'Hello, it's the taxman', *Government Computing* March: 20–21.

Burrows, B. (1994) 'The power of information: developing the knowledge based organization', *Long Range Planning* 27, 1: 142–51.

Cabinet Office (1999) *Modernising Government*, CM4310, London: Stationery Office.

Caldow, J. (1996) 'Reengineering government', *Government Computing International* October: 24–5.

Centrelink (1998) *Centrelink Annual Report 1997–98*, Canberra, Australia: Centrelink.

Centrelink (1999) *Centrelink Information: A Guide to Payments and Services, 1998–99*, Canberra, Australia: Centrelink.

Chapman, R. and Hunt, M. (1987) *Open Government*, London: Routledge.

Chatham House Forum (1998) *Open Horizons: Three Scenarios for 2020*, London: The Royal Institute of International Affairs.

Choo, C. (1996) 'The knowing organization: how organizations use information to construct meaning, create knowledge and make decisions', *International Journal of Information Management* 16, 5: 329–40.

Cleveland, H. (1985) 'The twilight of hierarchy: speculations on the global information hierarchy', *Information and Referral* 7, 1: 1–31.

Cross, M. (1998) *Healthsmart 2010: A Tale of Life, Death and Health Care in the Information Age*, London: Kable.

Crowston, K. and Malone, T. (1994) 'Information technology and work organization', in M. Scott Morton (ed.) *Information Technology and the Corporation of the 1990s*, Oxford: Oxford University Press.

Data Protection Registrar (1999) *Discussion of International Developments*, London: Data Protection Registrar. Available online http://www.open.gov.uk/dpr/summary.html (3 March 1999).

Davenport, T. (1996) *Think Tank*, Austin: University of Texas. Available online http://www.cio.com/cio (26 July 1998).

Davenport, T. and Prusak, L. (1998) *Working Knowledge: How Organizations Manage What They Know*, Cambridge, Mass.: Harvard Business School Press.

Davenport, T. and Short, J. (1990) 'The new industrial engineering: information technology and business process redesign', *Sloan Management Review* 31, 4: 11–27.

Davenport, T. and Stoddard, D. (1994) 'Reengineering: business change of mythic proportions?', *MIS Quarterly* June: 121–7.

Davidson, W. (1993) 'Beyond reengineering: the three phases of business transformation', *IBM Systems Journal* 32, 1: 65–79.

Denison, D. (1994) 'What is the difference between culture and climate?', *Journal of Management Science* 40, 1: 13–20.

Department for Social Security (1997) *Commonwealth Services Delivery Agency: Draft Policy Statement*, Canberra, Australia: Department for Social Security.

Department for Trade and Industry (1998) *Our Competitive Future: Building the Knowledge Driven Economy*, London: Stationery Office.

Dhillon, G. and Backhouse, J. (1996) 'Risks in the use of information technology within organisations', *International Journal of Information Management* 16, 1: 65–74.

Dixon, P. and John, D. (1989) 'Technology issues facing corporate management in the 1990s', *MIS Quarterly* September: 247–55.

Drucker, P. (1992) 'The new society of organizations', *Harvard Business Review* September/October: 6–20.

Due, R. (1995) 'The knowledge economy', *Information Systems Management* Summer: 76–8.

Dutton, W. (1996) *Information and Communication Technology*, Oxford: Oxford University Press.

Earl, M. (1995) *Information Equity: A Model for Measuring Performance in the Information Age*, Working Paper CRIM WP 96/2, London: London Business School.

Earl, M. and Sampler, J. (1998) 'Market management to transform the IT organization', *Sloan Management Review* Summer: 9–17.

Eaton, J. and Bawden, D. (1991) 'What kind of resource is information?', *International Journal of Information Management* 11, 2: 156–65.

Ellis, D. Barker, R. and Potter, S. (1993) 'Information audits, communication audits and information mapping: a review and survey', *International Journal of Information Management* 13, 2: 134–51.

Feather, J. (1998) *The Information Society: A Study of Continuity and Change*, London: Library Association.

Feeny, D. and Willcocks, L. (1998) 'Core IS capabilities for exploiting information technology', *Sloan Management Review* Spring: 9–21.

Fenton-O'Creevy, M. (1995) *Striking Off the Shackles: A Survey of Managers' Attitudes to Employee Involvement*, Corby: Institute of Management.

Fisher, A. (1998) 'Success secret: a high emotional IQ', *Fortune* October: 293–8.

Friedman, B. Hatch, J. and Walker, D. (1998) *Delivering on the Promise: How to Attract, Manage and Retain Human Capital*, New York: Free Press.

Galliers, R. (ed.) (1987) *Information Analysis: Selected Readings*, New York: Addison Wesley.

Garvin, D. (1993) 'Building a learning organization', *Harvard Business Review* July–August: 78–91.

Gerth, H. and Wright-Mills, C. (1958) *Max Weber: Essays in Sociology*, Oxford: Oxford University Press.

Glazer, R. (1993) 'Measuring the value of information: the information intensive organization', *IBM Systems Journal* 32, 11: 99–110.

Glazer, R. Steckel, J. and Winner, R. (1992) 'Locally rational decision making: the distracting effect of information on managerial performance', *Management Science* 38, 2: 212–26.

Goddard, T. and Riback, C. (1998a) *The Eight Traits of Highly Successful Public Officials*, Washington: The HILL. Available online http//www.youWon-NowWhat.com (10 April 1999).

Goddard, T. and Riback, C. (1998b) *You Won – Now What? How Americans Can Make Democracy Work from City Hall to the White House*, New York: Scribner.

Goleman, D. (1998) 'What makes a leader?' *Harvard Business Review* November–December: 93–102.

Grant, R. (1994) 'TQMs challenge to management theory and practice', *Sloan Management Review* Winter: 25–35.

Gross, N. (1995) 'The technology paradox', *Business Week* 6 March: 36–44.

Haak, T. and Lekanne Deprez, F. (1998) *Individual Balanced Scorecards: Capitalizing on Individual and Organizational Needs for Mutual Benefit*, Amsterdam, Netherlands: KPMG. Available online http://kpmg.interact.nl/publication-/publication.html (26 October 1998).

Haeckel, S. and Nolan, R. (1993) 'Managing by wirc', *Harvard Business Review* September–October: 122–32.

Hall, R. (1992) 'The strategic analysis of intangible resources', *Strategic Management Journal* 13: 135–44.

Hamel, G. and Prahalad, C. (1990) 'The core competencies of the corporation', *Harvard Business Review* May–June: 79–91.

Hamel, G. and Prahalad, C. (1994) 'Strategy as a field of study: why search for a new paradigm?', *Strategic Management Journal* 15, 6: 5–16.

Hammer, M. (1990) 'Reengineer work: don't automate, obliterate', *Harvard Business Review* July–August: 104–18.

Heeks, R. (1999) *Information Systems for the Public Sector: Working Paper Series No. 7*, Manchester: University of Manchester Institute for Development Policy and Management.

Hopper, M. (1990) 'Rattling SABRE – new ways to compete on information', *Harvard Business Review* May–June: 118–25.

Horovitz, J. (1984) 'New perspectives on strategic management', *Journal of Business Strategy* Winter: 19–33.

Horton, F. (1994) *Analyzing Benefits and Costs: A Guide for Information Managers*, Ottawa, Canada: International Development Research Centre.

Houdeshel, G. and Watson, H. (1987) 'Management information and decision support', *MIS Quarterly* March: 127–40.

Hsaio, R. and Ormerod, R. (1998) 'A new perspective on the dynamics of information technology enabled strategic change', *Information Systems Journal* June: 21–52.

IMPACT Ltd (1994) *Hawley Committee Report: Information as an Asset*, London: IMPACT Ltd.

Information security survey (1998) London: KPMG. Available online http://www.kpmg.co.uk/uk/services/irm/iss98/index.html (20 October 1998).

International Conference on Data Protection (1998) London: Data Protection Registrar. Available online http://www.open.gov.uk/dpr/20dpccom.html (3 March 1999).

ICA (International Council for Information Technology in Government Administration) (1998a) *Information Sharing Within and Between Governments*, Canberra, Australia: Office for Government Information Technology. Available online http://www.ogit.gov.au/ica/icaindex.html (24 February 1999).

ICA (International Council for Information Technology in Government Administration) *Discussion Reports* (1998b) Canberra, Australia: Office for Government Information Technology. Available online http://www.ogit.gov.au/ica/icaindex. html (26 October 1998).

Ireland, Department of Finance (1997) *Freedom of Information Act*, Dublin: Department of Finance.

Kaplan, R. and Norton, D. (1993) 'Putting the balanced scorecard to work', *Harvard Business Review* September–October: 134–47.

Keen, P. and Cummins, M. (1991) *Shaping the Future: Business Design through Information Technology*, Cambridge Mass.: Harvard Business School Press.

Kim, K. and Michelman, J. (1990) 'An examination of factors for the strategic use of information in the health care industry', *MIS Quarterly* 14, 2: 201–15.

Kotter, J. (1995) 'Leading change: why transformation efforts fail', *Harvard Business Review* September–October: 114–20.

Koulopoulos, T., Spinello, R. and Toms, W. (1997) *Corporate Instinct: Building a Knowledge Enterprise for the 21st Century*, New York: Van Nostrand Reinhold.

Kovacevic, A. and Majiluf, N. (1993) 'Six stages of IT strategic management', *Sloan Management Review* Summer: 77–87.

KPMG (1998a) *The Power of Knowledge*, London: KPMG. Available online http://www.kpmg.co.uk (14 January 1999).

KPMG (1998b) *Knowledge Management Research Report*, London: KPMG. Available online http://www.kpmg.co.uk (24 February 1999).

Lederer, A. and Sethi, V. (1992) 'Meeting the challenges of information systems planning', *Long Range Planning* 25, 2: 69–80.

Leonard-Barton, D. (1996) *Wellsprings of Knowledge: Building and Sustaining Sources of Innovation*, Cambridge, Mass.: Harvard Business School Press.

Lievesey-Howarth, R. (1997) 'Electronic governance: the risk to society', *The Australian*, 25 July, 32–3.

Luftman, J. (1993) 'Transforming the enterprise: the alignment of business and information technology strategies', *IBM Systems Journal* 32, 1: 198–221.

Malhotra, Y. (1997) 'Knowledge management in inquiring organizations', available online http:hsb.baylor.edu/ramsowee/ais.ac.97/papers/malhotr3html (8 May 1998).

Manasco, P. (1996) 'Information accounting systems', *Journal of Systems Management* June: 1–8.

Marchand, D. and Horton, F. (1986) *Infotrends: Profiting from your Information Resources*, New York: Wiley.

Massey, J. (1995) 'The information strategists', *Information Age* December: 30–5.

Matheson, S. (1997) 'Implementing an IT strategy: the UK Inland Revenue', in M. Earl (ed.) *Information Management: The Strategic Dimension*, Oxford: Clarendon Press, 202–9.

May, M. (1998) 'The new intangibles', *Information Strategy* 3, 6: 24–9.

Menou, M. (1993) *Measuring the Impact of Information on Development*, Ottawa, Canada: International Development Research Centre.

Milner, E. (1997a) 'Analysing the absence of information management in annual reports of FTSE listed company annual reports', unpublished research report, University of North London.

Milner, E. (1997b) 'Quality management, the right approach?', in J. Brockman (ed.) *Quality Management and Benchmarking in the Information Sector*, London: Bowker Saur.

Milner, E. (1999) 'Electronic government, more that just a good thing? A question of ACCESS', in B. Hague (ed.) *Digital Democracy*, London: Routledge.

Mintzberg, H. (1994) 'The fall and rise of strategic planning', *Harvard Business Review* January–February: 107–14.

Mori Ltd (1996) *Disconnect Research*, London: Mori Ltd.

National Health Service Executive (1998) *Information for Health: An Information Strategy for a Modern NHS 1998–2005*, London: National Health Service Executive.

Nonaka, I. (1991) 'The knowledge creating company', *Harvard Business Review* November–December: 96–104.

Nonaka, I. and Takeuchi, H. (1995) *The Knowledge Creating Company*, Oxford: Oxford University Press.

Orna, E. (1990) *Practical Information Policies: How to Manage Information Flows in Organisations*, Aldershot: Gower.

Orna, E. (1996) 'Information procedures and presentation in organisations: accident or design?', *International Journal of Information Management* 17, 4: 341–51.

Osborne, D. and Gaebler, T. (1992)*Reinventing Government: How the Entrepreneurial Spirit is Transforming the Public Sector*, Reading, Mass.: Addison Wesley.

Oxbrow, N. and Abell, A. (1999) *Investigation of Underpinning Skills for Knowledge Management: Training Implications*, London: TFPL.

Peters, T. (1992) *Liberation Management: Necessary Disorganization for the Nanosecond Nineties*, London: Macmillan.

Pinsonneault, A. and Kraemer, K. (1993) 'The impact of information technology on middle management', *MIS Quarterly* September: 271–92.

Pitroda, S. (1993) 'Development democracy, and the village telephone', *Harvard Business Review* November–December: 66–79.

Pollett, M. (1999) 'Ferreting out the benefit rules', *Government Computing* March: 28–9.

Porter, M. and Miller, V. (1985) 'How information gives you competitive advantage', *Harvard Business Review* July–August: 149–60.

Reith, P. (1997) *Towards a Best Practice Australian Public Service*, Canberra: Ministry for Industrial Relations.

Robson, W. (1997) *Strategic Information and Information Systems*, London: Pitman.

Rock, S. (1998) 'From the garden of Eden to the garden of Knowledge', *Journal of Business Strategy* Winter: 4–11.

Rowlands, I. (ed.) (1997) *Understanding Information Policy*, London: Bowker Saur.

Rutledge, R. (1997) 'The myths and mysteries of intellectual capital', *Strategic Management Journal* 28, 6: 9–17.

Schnitt, D. (1993) 'Reengineering the organization using information technology', *Journal of Systems Management* 44, 1: 14–20.

Scott Morton, M. and Allen, T. (1994)*Information Technology and the Corporation of the 1990s*, Oxford: Oxford University Press.

Senge, P. (1999) *The Dance of Change*, London: Nicholas Brealey.

Sparke, A. (1994) *A Practical Guide to Externalising Local Authority Services*, Harlow: Longman.

Stalk, G. (1988) 'Time, the next source of competitive advantage', *Harvard Business Review* July–August: 41–51.

Stewart, T. (1994) 'Your company's most valuable asset: intellectual capital', *Fortune* 3 October: 28–33.

Stewart, T. (1995) 'Mapping corporate brainpower', *Fortune* 30 October: 246–8.

Stewart. T. (1997) *Intellectual Capital: The New Wealth of Organizations*, New York: Currency/Doubleday.

Strassman, P. (1995) *The Politics of Information Management: Policy Guidelines*, Connecticut: Information Economics Press.

Sunday Times, Australia (1998) 15 November: 6.

Taylor, J. and Bellamy, C. (1998) *Governing in the Information Age*, Buckingham: Open University Press.

Teal, T. (1991) 'Services come first', *Harvard Business Review* September–October: 117–27.

Tebbutt, D. (1996) 'Drowning by numbers', *PC Pro* November: 224–9.

Thierauf, R. (1987) *A Problem Solving Approach to Effective Corporate Planning*, Westport, Conn.: Quorum.

Thornton, K. (1997) *Rethinking Government*, Washington: IBM.

Tissen, R. Andriessen, D. and Deprez, F. (1998) *Value-Based Knowledge Management*, London: Longman.

Tomlin, R. (1991) 'Developing a management culture in which IT can flourish: how the UK can benefit', *Journal of Information Technology* 6, 1: 45–55.

Torremans, P. and Holyoak, J. (1998) *Intellectual Property Law* 2nd edn, London: Butterworths.

Tozer, G. (1994) *Information Quality Management*, Manchester, Blackwell.

United Nations (1946) *Resolution of the United Nations General Assembly 59 (1)*, New York: 14 December.

Upton, R. and Swinden, K. (1998) *Think Global, Act Local, Government in the Information Age*, London: Kable.

Vardon, S. (1998) *Centrelink Community*, Canberra: Centrelink.

Vareljs, J. (1996) *Safeguarding Electronic Information*, Jefferson, NC: Mcfarland.

Venkatraman, N. (1994) 'IT-enabled business transformation: from automation to business scope redefinition', *Sloan Management Review* 35, 2: 74–88.

Watson, J. (1995) *Management Development to the Millennium: The New Priorities*, Corby: Institute of Management.

Westin, P. (1996) 'Data protection in the global society', unpublished proceedings of the American Institute for Contemporary German Studies workshop, 15 November.

White, M., Howells, A., Kibby, P. and Abell, A. (1998) *Intranet Management: A Guide to Best Practice*, London: TFPL.

Willcocks, L. (1993) *Information Systems in the Public Services: Management Trends and Issues in the United Kingdom*, Oxford: Institute of Information Management.

Willman, P. (1996) 'Protecting know-how', *London Business School Strategy Review* 7, 1: 9–13.

Wilson, I. (1992) 'Realising the power of strategic vision', *Long Range Planning* 25, 5: 18–28.

Zmud, R. (1986) 'The information economy: a new perspective', *Data Base* 2, 8: 17–23.

Index

ONE DIRECTION

SUPERSTARDOM!

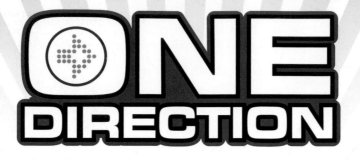

By Riley Brooks

D0107334

SCHOLASTIC

Photo credits:
Photographs © 2013:

AP Images: Cover foreground (Press Association); Back cover (Ian West/Press Association);
1 (Charles Sykes/Invision); 4 (Frank Micelotta/Invision); 21 (Owen Sweeney/Rex Features)

Corbis Images/Comic Relief/Splash News: 37

Getty Images: 8 (Larry Busacca); 12 (Craig Warga/NY Daily News); 16 (Mario Anzuoni/Reuters);
17 (Lucy Nicholson/Reuters); 18 (Myrna Suarez); 26 (Kenzo Tribouillard/AFP); 29 (Andreas Rentz);
30 (Franziska Krug); 31 (Jason LaVeris/FilmMagic); 33 (FOX)

45 (Kevin Mazur/WireImage), 48 (Tony Barson/WireImage)

Newscom: 38 (ZCVA WENN Photos); 41 (Hubert Boesl/dpa/picture-alliance);
42 (Matteo Bazzi/EPA)

Retna Ltd./Scott Weiner: 35

REX USA: 7 (Nikki To); 10; 22 (David Thompson); 40 & 47 (Brian Rasic); 43 (Ken McKay);
46 (Erik Pendzich)

Shutterstock, Inc./solarseven: Cover background

Splash News: 3; 15; 25 (Mercury Press)

© 2013 by Scholastic
ISBN 978-0-545-59131-7

Published by Scholastic Inc.
SCHOLASTIC and associated logos are trademarks and/or registered trademarks of
Scholastic Inc.

12 11 10 9 8 7 6 5 4 3 2 1   13 14 15 16 17 18/0

Printed in the U.S.A.   40
First printing, September 2013

Table of Contents

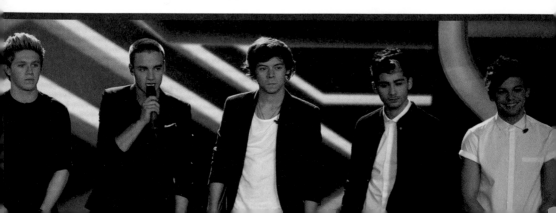

Introduction

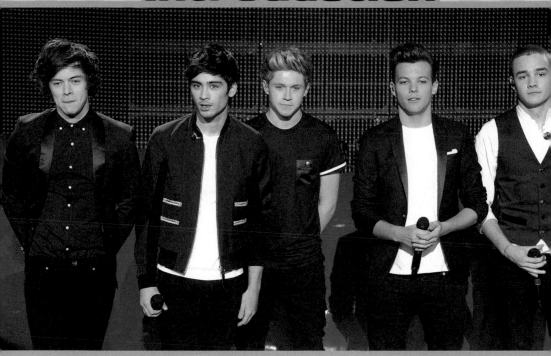

When they started off as contestants on the 2010 season of *The X Factor* in the UK, the guys of One Direction — Harry Styles, Liam Payne, Zayn Malik, Niall Horan, and Louis Tomlinson — had no idea that they would soon be a world-famous band. In fact, when they first auditioned for the reality

competition, it was as individuals competing *against* one another!

After the guys were each eliminated in the boot camp round, the *X Factor* judges suggested they form a group and continue in the competition. The rest of the show went really well for the newly formed One Direction. They even made it to the finals, and wound up taking home third place.

But third place wasn't enough for One Direction. Once they had a taste of what life was like in the spotlight, they wanted even more! Luckily, shortly after the conclusion of *The X Factor*, judge Simon Cowell offered the guys a recording contract. One Direction went right to work recording their first album, *Up All Night*, which would debut at number one in the US and go platinum. One Direction had gone from placing third on *The X Factor* in the UK to being the number-one band in America!

Welcome to the USA

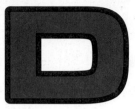uring 2012, One Direction spent a lot of time promoting *Up All Night* in the US. Their first US tour was as the opening act for Big Time Rush. The guys of BTR were as excited to be touring with One Direction as the 1D guys were to be taking the stage alongside Big Time Rush! Carlos Pena Jr. told MTV.com, "We are actually very similar on and off camera and we can't wait to have some fun on the road."

Even though BTR was very welcoming, the guys of One Direction were still nervous. They weren't sure American audiences would like them. But as soon as they took the stage, their fears flew out the window. Louis explained to Billboard.com, "We went onstage terrified that people would be like, 'Who are these blokes?' [But] we got an incredible reaction."

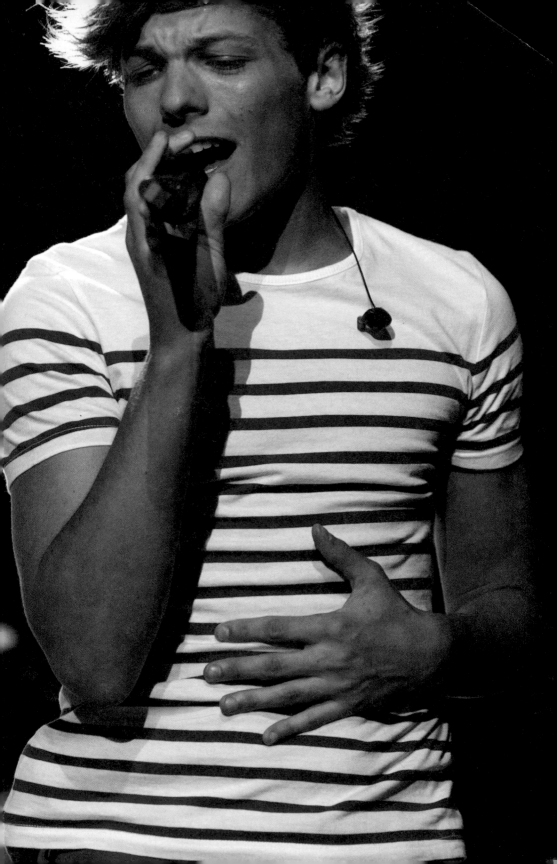

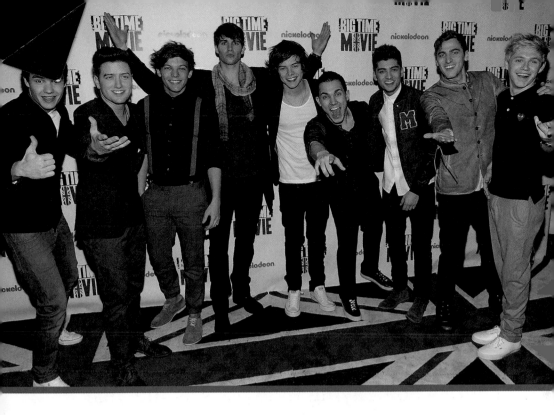

One Direction did not anticipate the kind of huge support they would get from their American fans. Louis told Billboard.com that he and the other guys were thrilled just to have the opportunity to tour the United States with Big Time Rush. "I remember we said as a band we would be really, really happy with a top 20 album—that would be incredible," he recalled. As luck would have it, though, while

One Direction was on tour with Big Time Rush, *Up All Night* hit number one on the charts, surpassing their expectations by miles.

Shortly after their successful tour with BTR, the guys were headlining their very own North American tour. Little did they know that less than a year later they would be headlining their own *world* tour! It was beyond their wildest dreams.

There's no denying it: 2012 was the year of One Direction. Harry, Louis, Liam, Zayn, and Niall went from being the opening act for Big Time Rush to having a number-one album in the US, a sold-out North American tour, and the spot as the most popular boy band in America. Lots of changes may have come their way since, but one thing is certain—One Direction is still on top!

CHAPTER 2
End of the Beginning

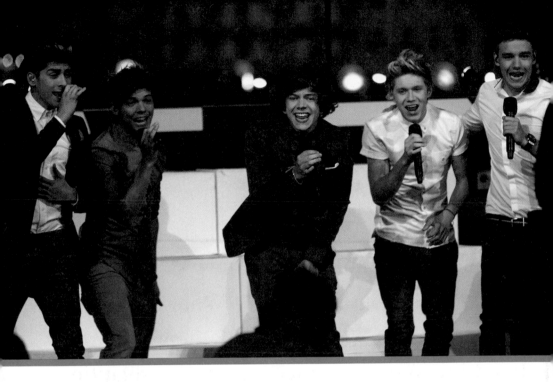

oward the end of 2012, the guys were invited to return to the UK to perform at the 2012 Summer Olympics in London. The closing ceremony was to include performers that best represented British culture. Among the other performers were Russell Brand, Jessie J, and the Spice

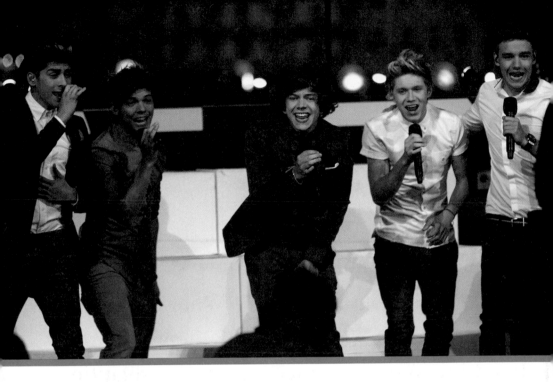

Girls. It was a huge honor for One Direction.

On August 12, 2012, One Direction performed during the closing ceremony of the Olympics to a packed crowd. Among the attendees were Prince Harry of England; Kate Middleton, Duchess of Cambridge; and One Direction's family members. "For me the Olympics literally can't be topped," Harry told Billboard.com. "The whole feeling was just unbelievable."

One Direction performed "What Makes You Beautiful" to a stadium full of cheering fans. In addition to the unique venue—a gigantic Olympic arena—the performance was unique in another way. The guys performed on a flatbed truck that drove them around the stadium as they sang. That's literally a *moving* performance! It was a fun night for all and a memorable one for the guys of 1D.

The next major British appearance for the

group was at the one hundredth anniversary of the Royal Variety Performance on November 19, 2012. This is an honor for any band since the show is for the royal family. The guys performed "Little Things" and even got to meet the Queen of England!

On December 3, 2012, the guys of One Direction found themselves back in the US, finishing off their North American tour with a sold-out concert at one of the most famous arenas in the United States—Madison Square

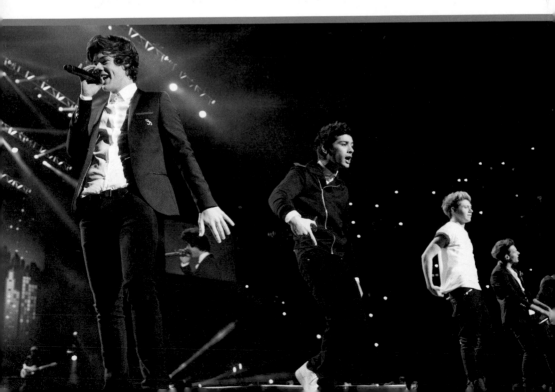

Garden. It was a chilly winter day, but fans from all over filled the stadium to see the guys. And 1D really appreciated the support. They even took questions from fans on Twitter and answered them during their performance!

Only four nights later on December 7, the band returned to the stage at Madison Square Garden to perform for a second time. This time it was as part of the radio station Z100's Jingle Ball. One Direction took the stage alongside fellow stars Justin Bieber, Taylor Swift, Ed Sheeran, and The Wanted. In an interview with Z100 DJ JJ, Harry talked about performing at Madison Square Garden. "I don't think you ever get tired of walking into that room," he said. Not only can One Direction say they headlined Madison Square Garden, they can say they played there twice in one week!

Awesome Awards

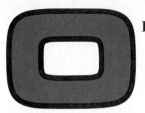ne Direction is an international sensation, so it's no surprise that they've won awards in countries all over the world, including Australia, Mexico, Germany, Japan, and Brazil.

In America, One Direction was nominated three times at the 2012 MTV Video Music Awards. The most important nomination was for Best New Artist, which Justin Bieber and Lady Gaga have both won in the past. The guys knew that taking home this award would definitely be a huge win for them and their fans. The guys faced some stiff competition against other amazing newcomer artists like fun. and Carly Rae Jepsen. But ultimately, One Direction snagged the prize along with awards for Best Pop Video (which they won over Justin Bieber) and Most Share-worthy Video.

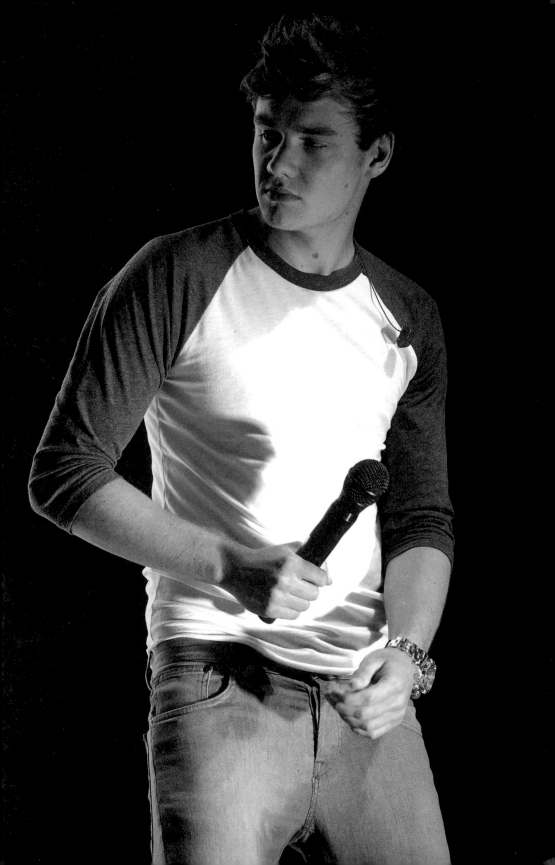

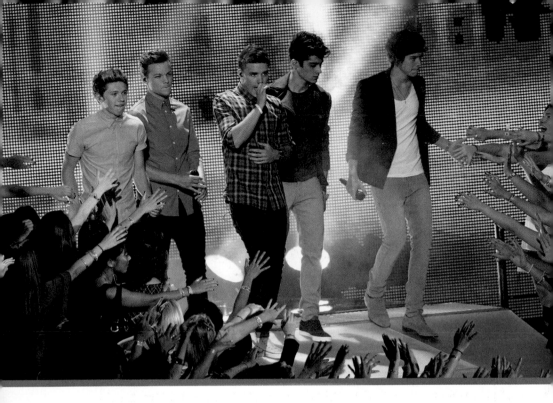

Aside from being nominees that night, One Direction was also slated to perform at the awards show for the first time ever. Liam told MTV.com, "I think performing at the VMAs is such a huge occasion. I think it ranks up there with one of the best performances we'll do so far." Fans were really excited to see what One Direction's first MTV VMA performance would be like, and they were not disappointed. One Direction performed "One Thing" to a

screaming crowd and had everyone singing along.

The importance of the performance was not lost on the guys. Harry told Billboard.com, he felt like people learned a bit more what the band is all about from their performance. "To be on that stage and perform was unbelievable," he said.

One Direction had a really successful night with both their awesome performance and the awards they took home. But they never lost sight of why they were there in the first place—it was thanks to their amazing fans.

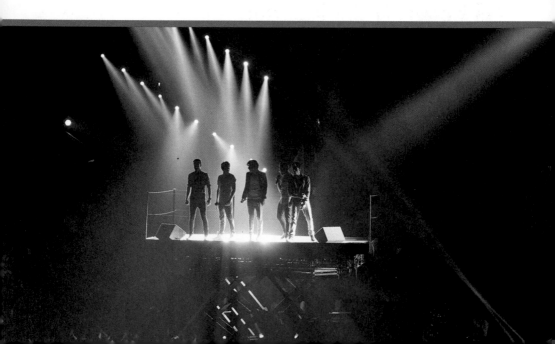

Back in the Studio

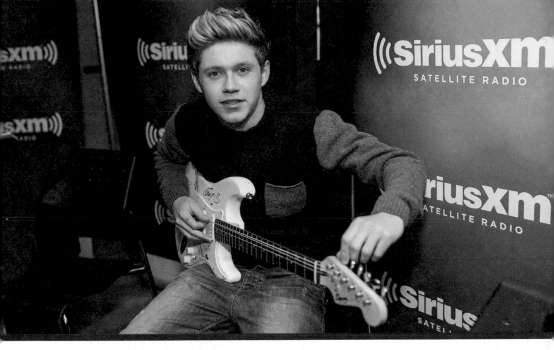

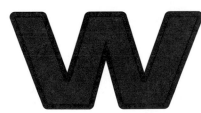ith everything they accomplished in 2012, it's hard to believe One Direction also recorded their second album, *Take Me Home*, that same year. Because of their jam-packed tour schedule, the guys only had about a month in the studio during the summer to record the album.

With such a short window of recording time, the guys had to make sure each song was right for them. Harry told NPR.org, "The thing with this album was it was so quick; we had so little time. We recorded everything in about a month, and it was at the point where we couldn't waste time doing songs if we didn't like them and didn't think they were going to [go anywhere]."

During the recording process, the guys had a lot more input on this album than they had on their first one. They were more involved with the songwriting, and they were able to really give fans what they wanted while exploring their personal musical tastes. Harry told DJ Nick Grimshaw, host of a BBC Radio 1 show, that he thought the band's experience helped them record even better songs than those on their first album.

With five band members, the group needed

to work together to come up with music that had the One Direction feel to it. Liam told Billboard.com that he and the others usually worked in smaller groups. "When you have more than two people working together it gets a bit unfocused....We tend to pair off a little bit," he recalled.

The guys had a really great team working with them as well. A lot of the people who worked on *Up All Night* were back collaborating with One Direction again for the second album. Niall told Teen.com, "We just kind of sit in a room, and we're lucky enough to work with some really great songwriters, so we just chill and then someone comes up with an idea. Then we just go cracking on that, then I get out the guitar and play some chords, and then we just write the track afterwards."

With more input on the songwriting, the album's success depended on how much work

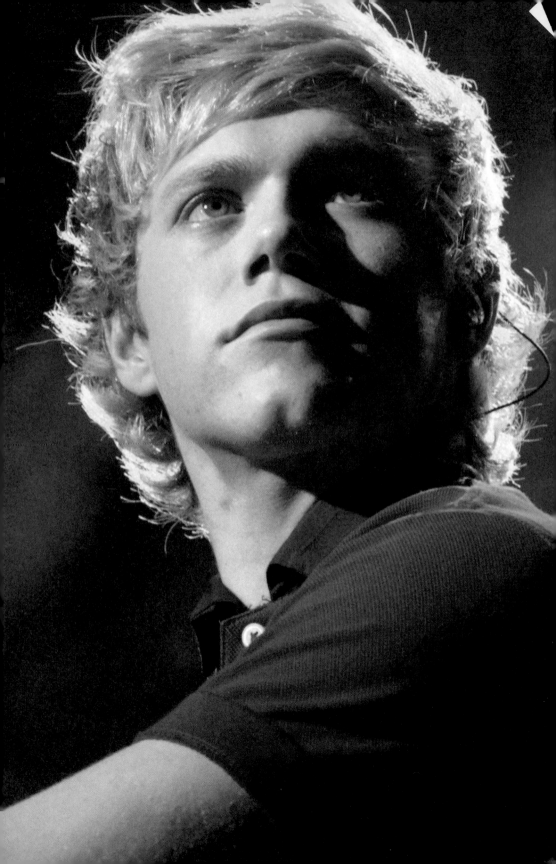

the guys put into it, which added some pressure. The guys wondered if they could possibly top the success of *Up All Night*. Even though the band had poured their hearts into the new album, they were unsure of how fans and critics would receive it. In an interview at the 2012 iTunes Festival, Harry said, "Everyone's said that second albums are the hardest, so before we started recording we were a bit nervous."

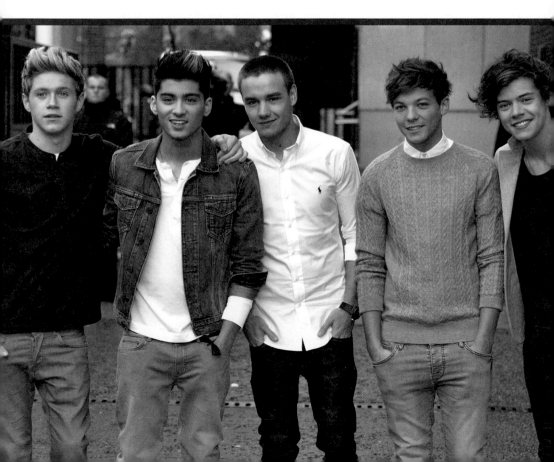

As for the album name, all the guys made sure they were involved in that as well. Niall told *On Air with Ryan Seacrest* that he and the others got together and thought about it for a while. "We all . . . do a lot of traveling around the world and we get to see a lot of cool places, but the main thing is there's no place like home," Niall explained.

On November 9, 2012, the guys' hard work paid off when they released their sophomore album, *Take Me Home*. The guys knew that they had another number-one album on their hands. In the first week, it amazingly sold 540,000 copies, making it the third-fastest selling album of the year (Taylor Swift's *Red* and Mumford & Sons' *Babel* took first and second, respectively). One Direction had done it again!

Take Me Home

About a month after the release of *Take Me Home*, the album had sold a million copies, solidifying it as a platinum hit. Niall told Seventeen.com, "We've worked really hard to get the music right and try to make it better than the last one. I think you can expect it to be really fun—the songs make everyone happy. They will make you smile."

In order to get fans excited for their new album, One Direction actually released their first single, "Live While We're Young," a little earlier than the album. The track sold so many copies before the album was even released that it was the fastest-selling pre-order single of all time. It was also featured in a Pepsi television commercial starring the guys of 1D and Super Bowl-winning quarterback Drew Brees of the

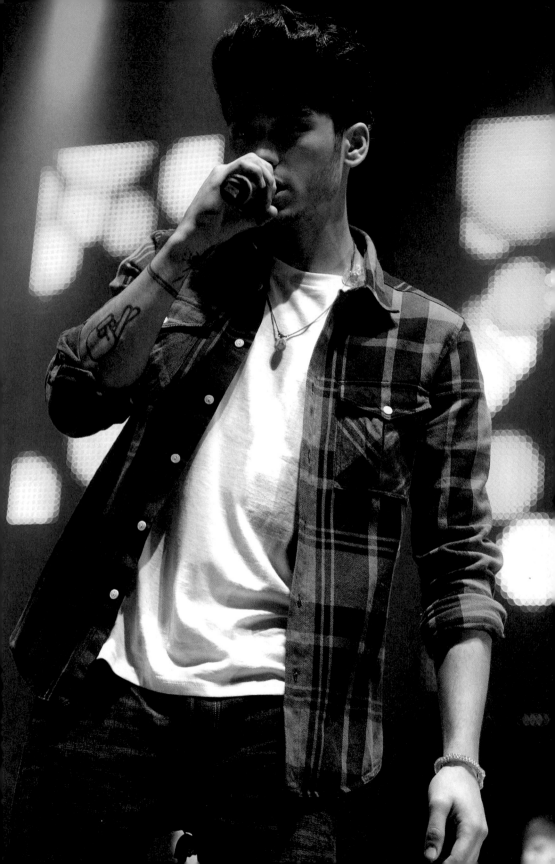

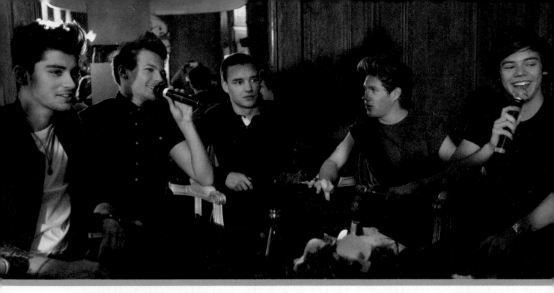

New Orleans Saints. In the US, Drew Brees may be a celebrity, but most of the guys had no clue who he was before they met him on the commercial shoot! "Honestly...American football is not that big over in the UK, so we hadn't really heard of Drew Brees before," Zayn told Billboard.com. "I did know that he was, like, a massive football player...so I was still a little bit anxious and nervous to meet him. I think Niall knew who he was. He was a really cool guy and quite funny....We just had a lot of fun on that Pepsi shoot."

As their second single off the album, the

band released "Little Things," which was written by Ed Sheeran. The acoustic song was quite different than any of One Direction's previous singles. Niall told Billboard.com, "It's broadening the audience for sure.... It's great for opening people up at our shows. As you know, a lot of our TV performances are quite high energy. We want to just sit down and sing the song and show people what we are [all about]."

After "Little Things," One Direction went right back to what their fans love them most for—pop—with the song "Kiss You." Not only were fans delighted by the song, One Direction was, too! Liam told MTV.com, "With the album, that's the first one that we listened to and we were like, 'Yeah, we love this song.' It holds a special place in our [hearts]."

The band's love of this song comes through in the fun music video they filmed for it. "I

think the whole concept behind the video is bigger than anything we've done before," Zayn told MTV.com.

But recording the video wasn't all fun and games. It still took a lot of team effort and planning. Liam told MTV.com, "There were proper sets and everything for this video, and there was a lot of hard work that went into it with the crew and everything." As if the "Kiss You" video isn't epic enough with its major costume changes and background swaps, the guys filmed it on a truly epic stage. "We shot it where *Star Wars* was shot on the George Lucas stage," Niall revealed to MTV.com.

None of the One Direction guys could have anticipated the huge success of *Take Me Home*. With the release of *Up All Night*, the guys were the first British group to debut at number one in the US. Now, with *Take Me Home*, the guys had achieved yet another

record. They became the first group to have two albums in one year makc the top five on the end-of-the-year chart.

After releasing *Take Me Home*, the guys set out on their first world tour as headliners beginning in February 2013. The tour kicked off in London, and from there the guys performed in countries all over the world, including Germany, Portugal, Spain, Italy, France, Mexico, Australia, and Canada. And, of course, the guys headed back to the US for part of their tour.

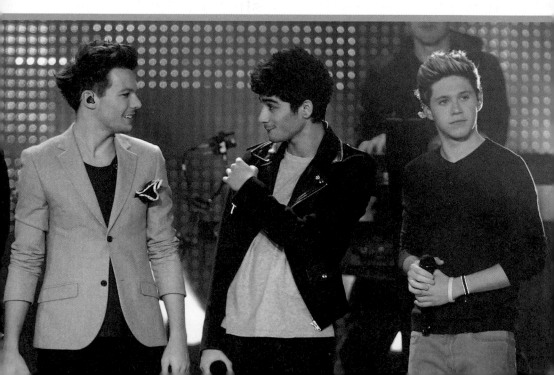

Just the Guys

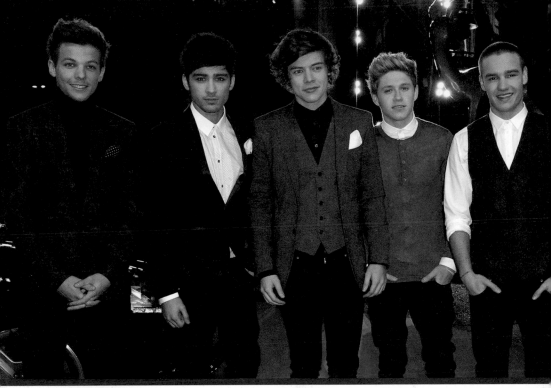

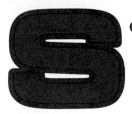o, what exactly is it like behind the scenes with 1D? It's definitely all about fun and friendship. Even though the guys started out as strangers when they were on *The X Factor*, they are now best buds. After all, they spend almost every day together!

Because of all the time they've spent working and playing together, the guys have become like brothers and are always there to support one another. Louis told Seventeen.com, "Harry is the guy I can really talk to about anything, but I love to have a heart-to-heart with Zayn as well. And if I'm going to run off and do something crazy, I would choose Liam. He's so carefree and easygoing."

The guys spend a lot of time with one another in close quarters—like their tour bus. Louis told Seventeen.com that to pass the time

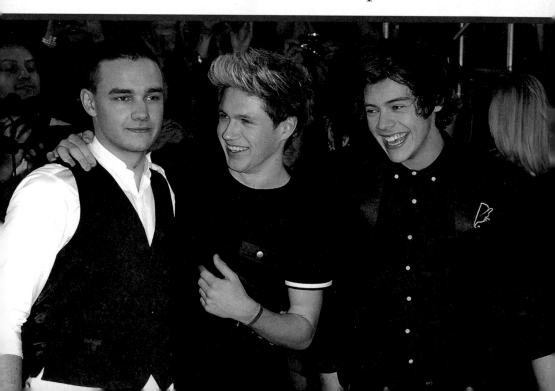

on long trips "We play cards, Playstation, chat with each other, and watch movies." Plus the guys love to play pranks on one another.

Aside from hanging out with one another, the guys have been known to hang out with other famous faces. They often find themselves in the recording studio with Ed Sheeran. They bump into Justin Bieber backstage and in day-to-day life. Niall and Justin even Tweeted a picture of themselves making dinner together! Niall is also very friendly with Demi Lovato. Niall told Seventeen.com, "She has a fantastic attitude. If I ever needed anything or needed to talk to anybody, I think Demi would be the person to talk to." Demi also had something to say about Niall. She told Seventeen.com, "I think Niall is super, super sweet and we've become good friends. I get what it's like to be in the spotlight since I've grown up in it."

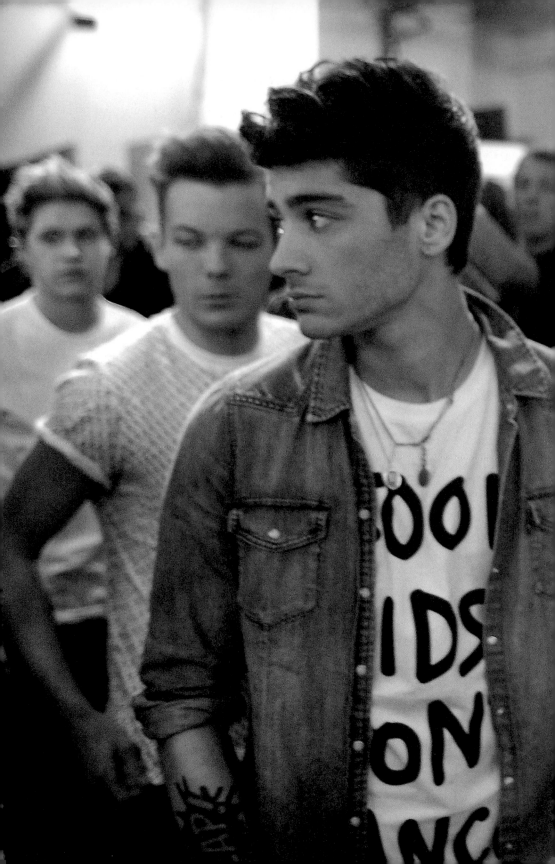

When it comes to the holidays, the guys look forward to relaxing with family and friends since they are always on the go during the year. Niall told MTV.com his favorite thing about Christmas is spending it with family and friends, eating a lot, and chilling out. That sounds a lot like any other guy!

The guys may seem like they're always cool, calm, and collected, but they still have their embarrassing moments.

"One time Harry and I were skiing together when a girl and a guy came up to us with a camera," Louis told Seventeen.com. "We assumed they were going to ask us for a photo, so we stood there with our arms around each other, posing. They said, 'No, we want *you* to take a photo of *us*!' It was embarrassing!"

And believe it or not, even though the guys have played a lot of shows, including two at Madison Garden, they still get nervous! Niall

told DigitalSpy.com, "When we first started out, the thought of getting up on stage freaked us all out. The kinds of crowds we get are very, very loud which helps. The bigger the crowd the better, really! The noise calms your nerves."

When it comes down to it, the band is just five ordinary guys doing amazing things. They get to travel the world and meet awesome people, but they really are just regular guys at heart!

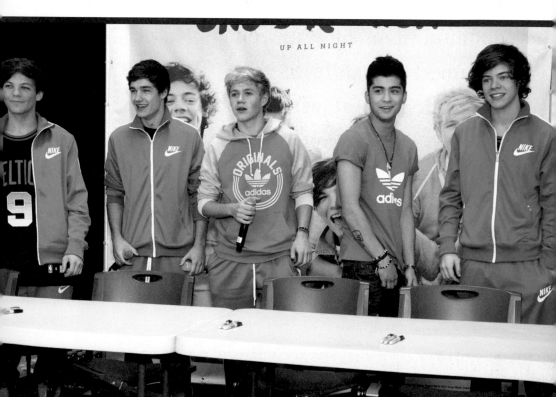

Giving Back

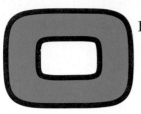ne Direction is so thankful for all of their success and knows that their fans are the reason why they are where they are today. The guys are always looking to give back to their fans, no matter how packed their schedules may be.

One Direction has worked with Rays of Sunshine, a group that grants wishes to children in need. The guys visited with some kids associated with the organization and donated their time. Liam told TheSun.co.uk, "It's such a small thing for us but the kids get so much out of it. We really love doing things like this. We leave smiling because they are always so wonderful." Niall also added, "It is totally humbling to meet kids like this. And it really makes you feel good that you can do something nice for them. We've had amazing

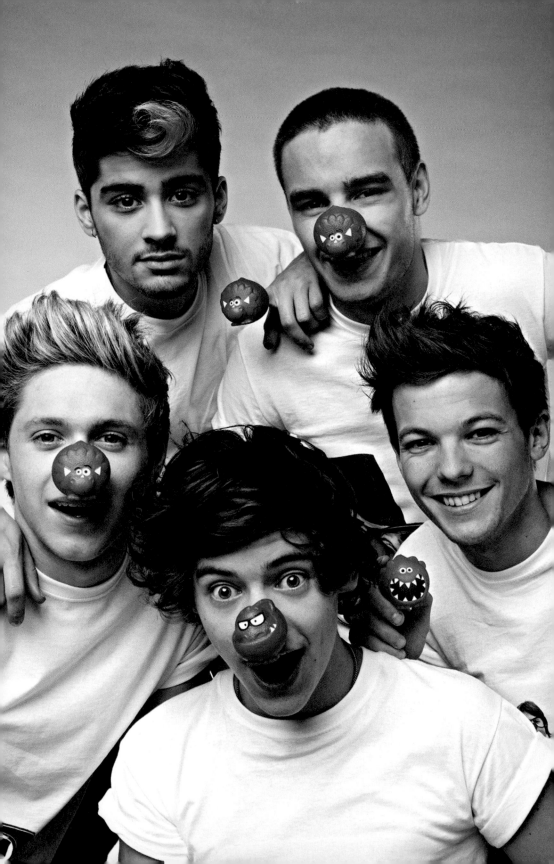

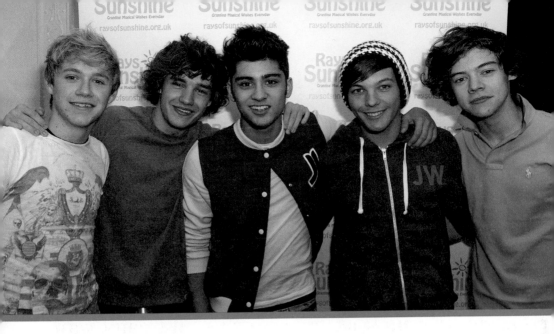

good luck and many of these children haven't. But they are always happy and we go away feeling brilliant. It's like we're giving something back." One Direction didn't stop there, though. They also donated a recipe for the Rays of Sunshine *Dish for a Wish Cookbook* to raise more funds for the organization.

The guys also recorded the official single for the British charity Comic Relief. The single is the band's version of the song "One Way Or Another," which was originally performed by Blondie. The guys also participated in a

telethon for Comic Relief called Red Nose Day. This cause was one the guys definitely knew they wanted to be a part of.

Harry told TheSun.co.uk, "We have grown up with Comic Relief and taken part in lots of Red Nose Days at school so we were thrilled to be asked to do this year's Red Nose Day single. It's such an honor for us. We can't wait to perform our version of this iconic pop song and raise as much money as possible for this incredibly important cause that is really close to our hearts."

As part of their involvement with Red Nose Day, the guys also took a trip to Accra, Ghana, to visit with some children in need at a school. The guys of One Direction are always happy to give back to their communities. They know that their charitable works have a lot of influence in the world and they want to use that influence for good.

1D in 3-D

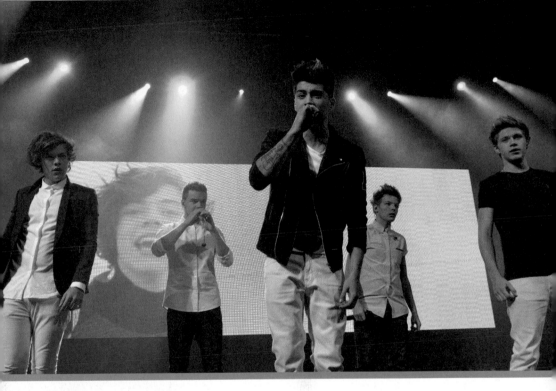

Haven't had a chance to see 1D live yet? Well, you're in luck. The guys have just released a 3-D concert movie. Niall told MTV.com that the band was filmed every day during their 2012 American tour. And Louis promised fans an intimate look at his fellow bandmates. "We've

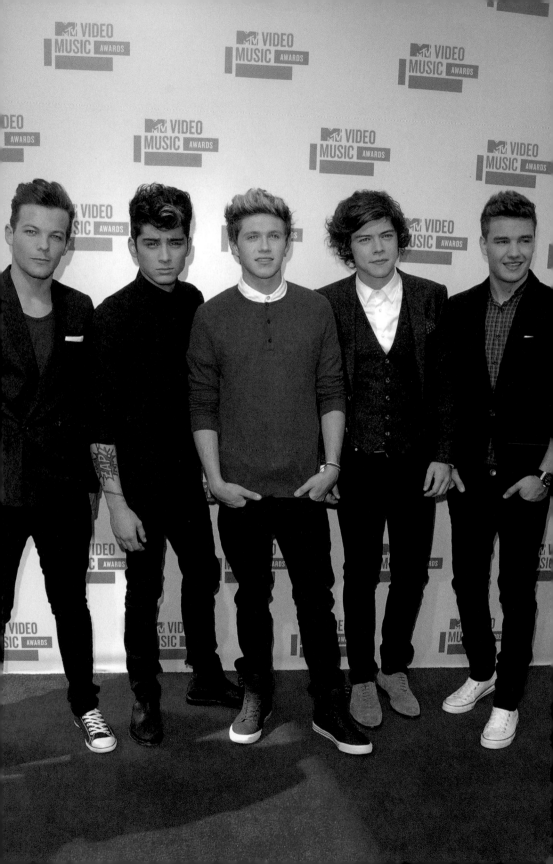

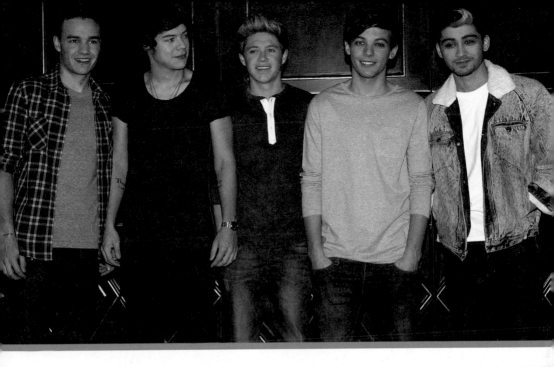

been documenting stuff for a long time, actually, just because it's important," he told Billboard. com. "I'm really excited about the...film, it's a great chance to all get across our personalities. The fans do know them to a degree, but they'll get a real chance to have a real insight on what our day to day is and exactly what we do."

Just like with their music, the guys wanted to be as involved as possible with the movie. In fact, Niall recorded some of the film with his own camera! One Direction also worked

with Academy Award-nominated director Morgan Spurlock of *Supersize Me* fame. "Morgan works well because...he did a lot of documentary movies," Niall told MTV. com. "That's more so what we want our movie to be. It's going to be a concert movie, but with a documentary side...."

If you haven't seen the movie yet, keep an eye out for it at a movie theater near you!

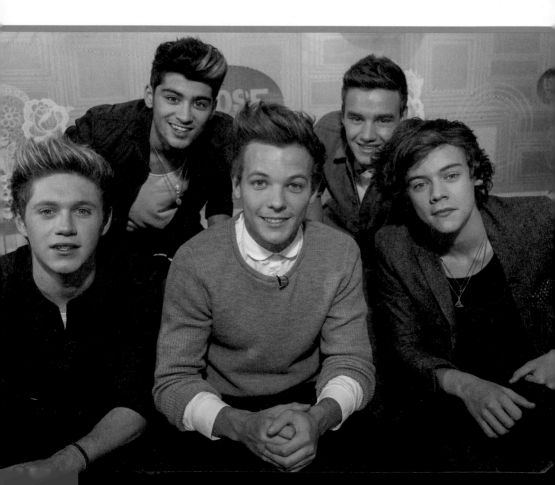

What's Next?

The kind of success 1D has had in just a year really only happens to a few lucky people. And of course there are other performers out there who want it just as badly as they do. Many interviewers ask the guys about their vision of the future, and whether the guys of 1D think they can have long-term success, given the history of other similar boy bands. In response, Liam told Billboard.com, "We know that this won't last forever, but we're having a great time out here. It's just amazing . . . It's just about living in this moment."

The kind of instant fame that 1D has achieved in 2012 could easily go to a guy's head. But the guys of One Direction are trying to remain focused and down-to-earth, with an eye toward the future. And the thought of

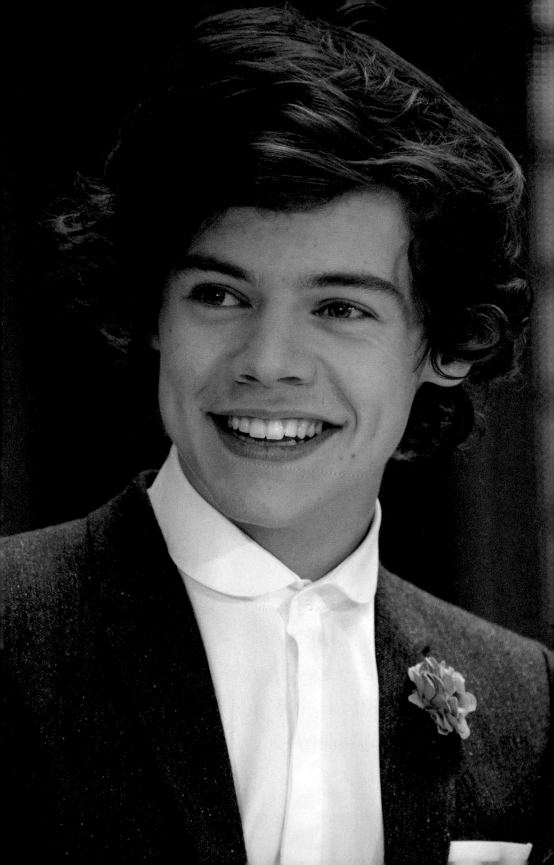

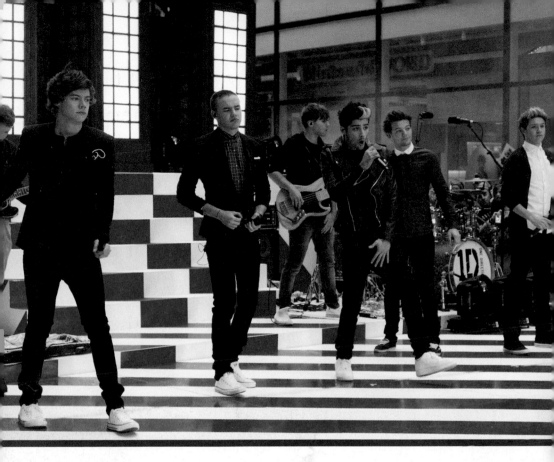

letting something they so quickly gained slip through their fingers is a scary thought. "I think it is important that we kind of keep our heads screwed on and keep looking forward," Harry told NPR.org.

Well, 1D better get ready for a whirlwind! Their third album, *Where We Are*, will be available by Christmas 2013. And what

better way to celebrate than with a worldwide stadium tour that kicks off in Latin America in the spring of 2014? At the UK press conference to announce the tour, Harry said, "It's going to be a completely different show from the *Take Me Home* tour. It's going to be much bigger. It's going to be a lot of fun. I can't wait." And eager 1D fans across the globe can't wait, either!

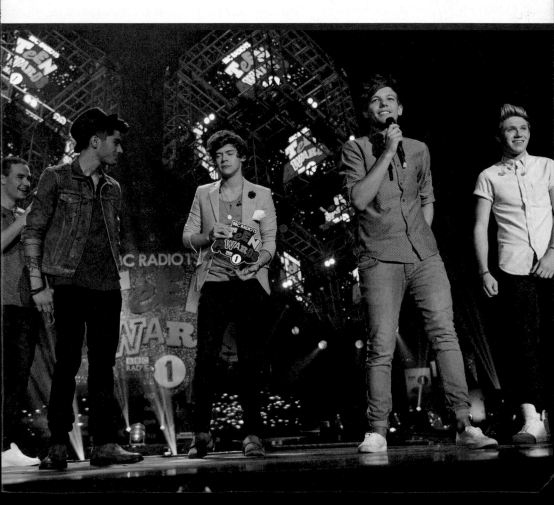

1D Online

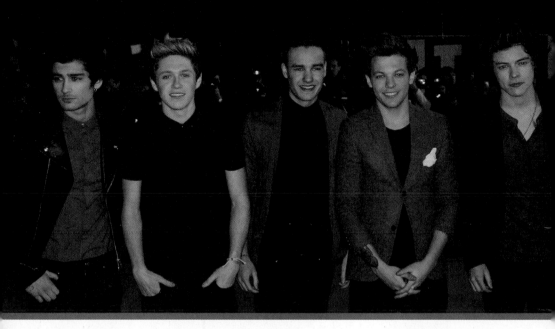

Want more info on One Direction?
Check out their official sites:

Official Website:
www.onedirectionmusic.com

Official Twitter:
@onedirection

Official Facebook:
www.facebook.com/onedirectionmusic